Book of Hope

AF006098

Book of Hope

Healthcare and Survival in the North

STORIES COLLECTED BY
AGNES R. PASCAL

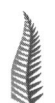

Fernwood Publishing
Halifax & Winnipeg

Copyright 2025 © Agnes R. Pascal

All rights reserved. No part of this book may be reproduced or transmitted in any form by any means without permission in writing from the publisher, except by a reviewer, who may quote brief passages in a review.

Development editor: Fazeela Jiwa
Copyediting: Brenda Conroy
Text design: Lauren Jeanneau
Cover design: Jess Koroscil
Printed and bound in the UK

Published by Fernwood Publishing
Halifax and Winnipeg
2970 Oxford Street, Halifax, Nova Scotia, B3L 2W4
www.fernwoodpublishing.ca

Fernwood Publishing Company Limited gratefully acknowledges the financial support of the Government of Canada through the Canada Book Fund and the Canada Council for the Arts. We acknowledge the Province of Manitoba for support through the Manitoba Publishers Marketing Assistance Program and the Book Publishing Tax Credit. We acknowledge the Nova Scotia Department of Communities, Culture and Heritage for support through the Publishers Assistance Fund.

This project was made possible, in part, with funding from the Government of the Northwest Territories and Hotıı̀ ts'eeda.

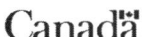 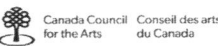 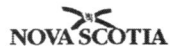 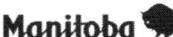

Library and Archives Canada Cataloguing in Publication
Title: Book of hope : healthcare and survival in the North / stories collected by Agnes R. Pascal.
Other titles: Book of hope (2025)
Names: Pascal, Agnes R., compiler.
Identifiers: Canadiana 20250142147 | ISBN 9781773637365 (softcover) | ISBN 9781773637921 (hardcover)
Subjects: LCSH: Rural health services—Canada, Northern. | LCSH: Cancer—Patients—Care—Canada, Northern. | LCSH: Indigenous peoples—Medical care—Canada, Northern.
Classification: LCC RA771.7.C3 B66 2025 | DDC 362.1/0425709719—dc23

To all those touched by cancer across the North and in memory of all those who fought a good fight while here on earth.

To Ister (Velma), David, Stephen, and Florence, who greatly touched our lives with strength, courage, and love, mahsi.

To my greatest blessing, my jijuu (grandmother) Laura Pascal. You planted the seed of faith within me with your unconditional love; with that foundation of faith I can overcome mountains. I love you and miss you every day, mahsi for your love.

To my dear brother Alfred Moses, for your presence and support in my journey of life and for all you were and are to my children Ronnie and Laura, mahsi and all our love.

Until we all meet again on that beautiful shore, we will forever carry each of you in our hearts, never to be forgotten.

Contents

MORE THAN YOU'LL EVER KNOW 1
Danita Frost-Arey

MAPS 2

THESE STORIES MATTER 4
Katłà (Catherine) Lafferty, Sara Komarnisky & Agnes Pascal

STORIES 16

Kátł'odeeche (Hay River)
    Annie Firth-Jones 16
    Kelsey Townend (McGinley) 22

Tindeè/Tu Nedhé (Great Slave Lake)
    Catherine Boucher 25
    James (Jim) Lynn 28
    Toni Anderson 30
    Elizabeth (Sabet) Biscaye 36
    Stephen Buchanan 44
    Allice Legat 46
    Patrick Scott 57
    Rueben Unka 64
    Lianne Mantla-Look 68
    Cecilia Rabesca 73

Deh Cho (MacKenzie River)
    Florence Barnaby 78
    Melinda Laboucan 84

Teetł'it Gwinjik (Peel River)

- Grace Martin 90
- Agnes Pascal 94
- Mary Effie Snowshoe 102
- Elizabeth Vittrekwa 107
- Ernest Vittrekwa 114
- Alice Vittrekwa 120
- Maria Ellen Voudrach (Peterson) 123

Nagwichoonjik/Kuukpak (Mackenzie River)

- Charlie Furlong 126
- Kirsten Fleuty 132
- Sandra Lynn Malcolm 139
- Winston Moses 145
- Ashley Wendland 149
- Ruth Wright 153

Nunaryuam Qaangani Tariuq (Arctic Ocean)

- Clara Bates 159
- Anonymous 163

ADVICE AND ACTIONS FROM STORYTELLERS 170

ACKNOWLEDGEMENTS 175

More Than You'll Ever Know

DANITA FROST-AREY

She said, "I'll fight until the very end
I'll show them how strong I really am
There's nothing God won't help me through."
Well Mom, I'll always be here for you
I love you more than you'll ever know
your love is one I'll never outgrow
your heart is where I find home
Mom, you're never really alone
She said, "I'll fight until the very end
I'll show them how strong I really am
there's nothing God won't help me through."
Well Mom, I'll be here to help you too
cause I love you more than you'll ever know
your love is one I'll never outgrow
and your heart is where I find home
and that's something I've always known
And then she said, "I love you my girls
I'd love to give you the whole world
cause I love you more than you'll ever know
regardless of how much you've grown
and I'll fight until the very end
I'll show them how strong I really am
and there's nothing God won't help me through."

Beaufort Delta Landscape. Photo by Eighty-One Images.

2 / BOOK OF HOPE

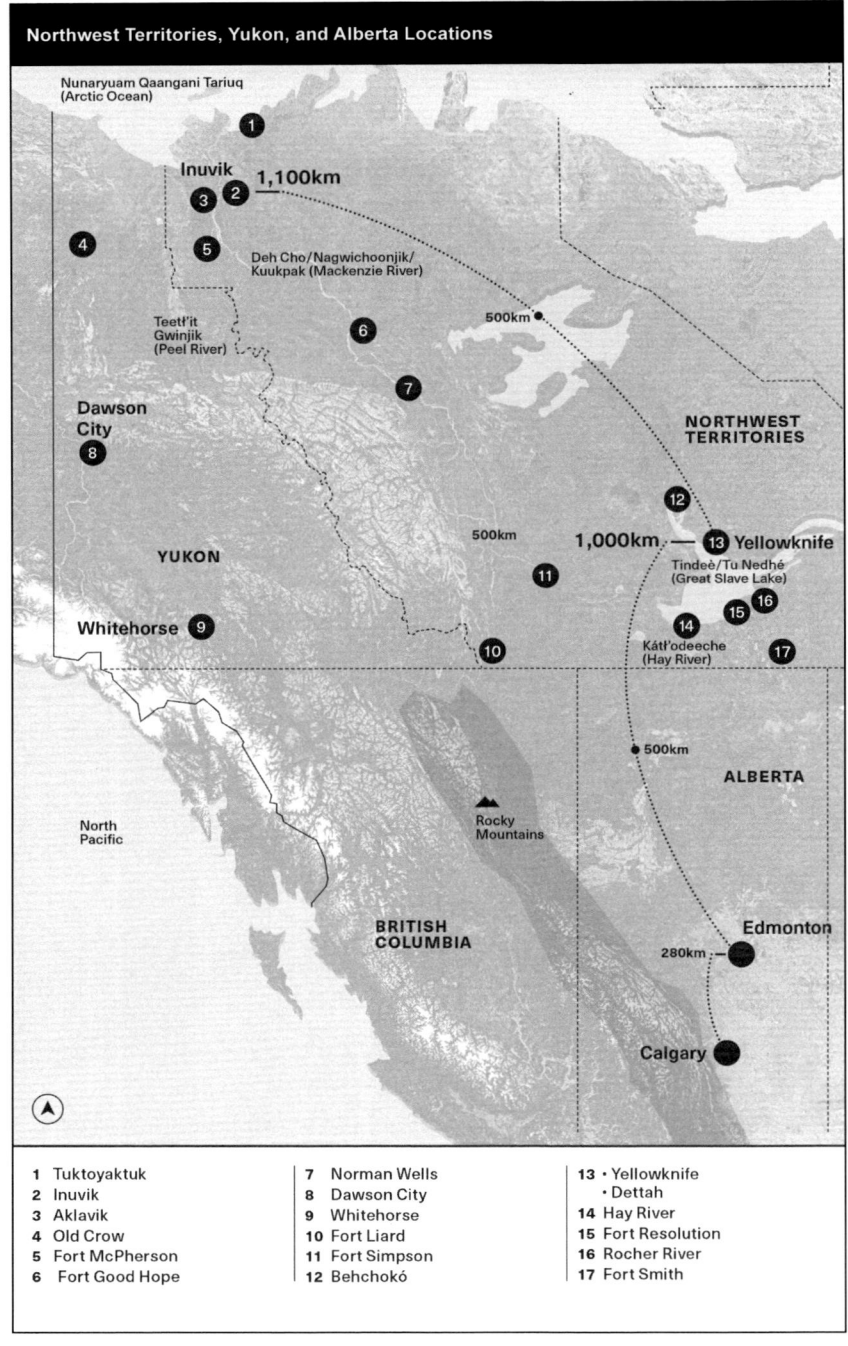

Map of NWT, Yukon, and Alberta Locations. Created by Evan Marnoch.

Maps / 3

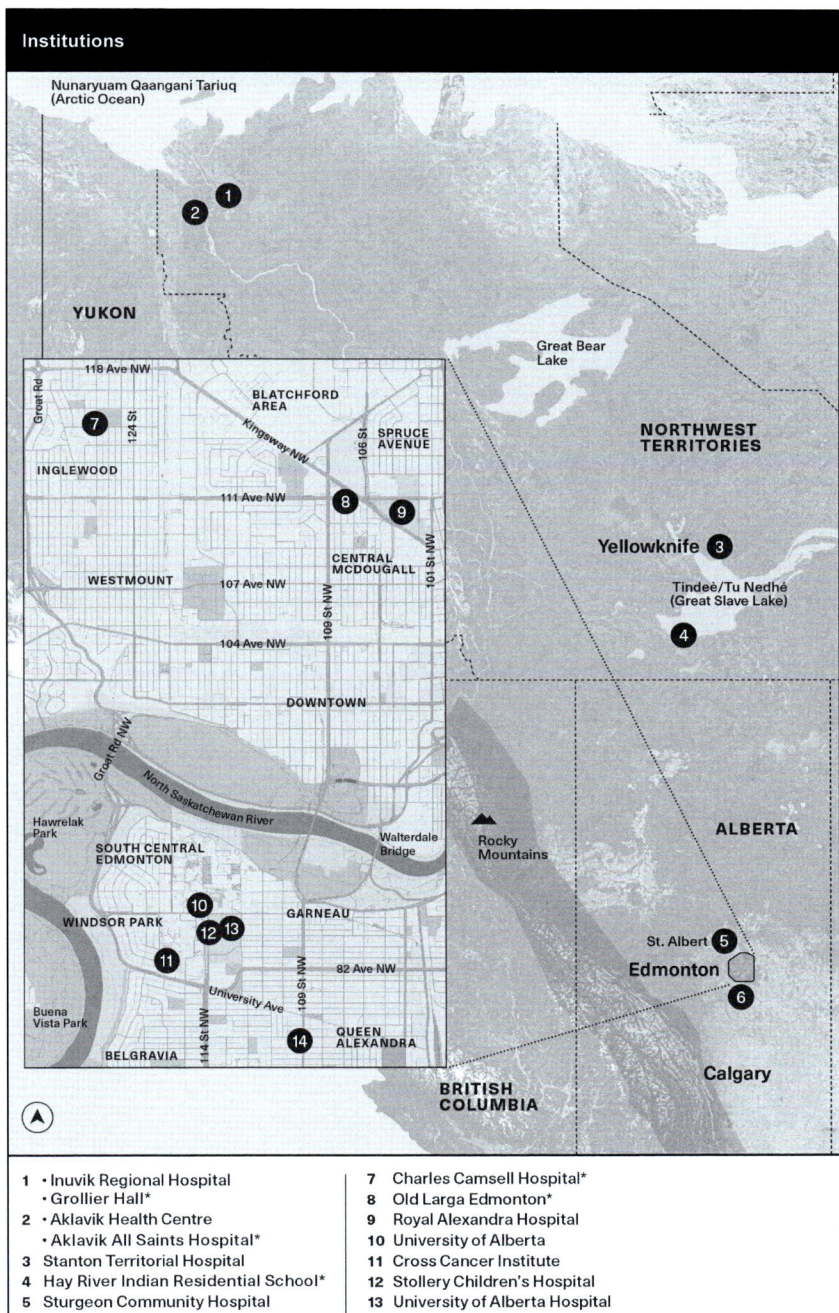

Map of NWT, Yukon, and Alberta Locations. Created by Evan Marnoch.

These Stories Matter

KATŁJÀ (CATHERINE) LAFFERTY, SARA KOMARNISKY & AGNES PASCAL

Across the North families experience anxious anticipation when a loved one is in peril. They sit together for long hours in waiting rooms. They lose sleep. They don't eat. They search for answers. When our loved ones are flown down South for medical care and we can't be with each other in those times of need, we feel powerless. When things feel completely out of our control, we worry. We pray for a miracle. Above all, we hope. We hope that there is, just for once, some fairness in a world that seems to have no mercy. Many of us, if given the chance, would opt to live longer and do things differently if we had more time. Many of the contributors in this book teach us that we shouldn't wait until we hear the dreaded word "cancer" to start living.

This book is special. It has been carefully crafted since the idea first stemmed from the stories shared by participants in the Inuvik Cancer Support Group. It has been a community-driven effort created as a source of hope for readers who may be going through similar cancer journeys. *Book of Hope* storytellers take us through their experiences from diagnosis, to travel from remote communities, to challenges in navigating it all. We hope this book shows Northern cancer

Katłįà (Catherine) Lafferty, Agnes Pascal, and Sara Komarnisky. Photo by Adze Studios/Amos Scott.

patients and their caregivers and family members that they are not alone and that their stories matter.

The Geography of Care

The Northwest Territories extends from the border with Alberta and Saskatchewan in the south, all the way to Borden Island in the Arctic Ocean. To the east is Nunavut, and to the west is Yukon. Approximately 45,000 residents live in 33 communities, ranging in size from the capital city, Yellowknife, at approximately 19,000 people, to Kakisa, with a population of 36. We are one of only two jurisdictions in Canada with a majority Indigenous population (the other is Nunavut), and twelve communities have no all-season road access. Our territory is rich and diverse in culture and language. Eleven languages are recognized here, eight of which are Indigenous.[1] We have a unique governance landscape, with historical treaties, modern treaties, Indigenous governments, and land claims currently in process — as well as settler governments at the federal, territorial, and municipal levels.

It is generally agreed that our people were strong and healthy prior to colonization. Dene oral history teaches about the wealth and health experienced by those living a customary life on the land:

> Berries, poplar sap, wild carrots … beaver meat, wild chicken, fish, anything, all those were eaten, that is why the people on the land were strong. Even though it was 40 below it did not bother anyone. Even though it was cold, children had their snowshoes on and were all over the place. They used to live strong and healthy.
>
> — Johnny Klondike, Dene Elder[2]

Inuvialuit, Dene, Métis, and Cree Peoples in this region have drawn on land-based medicine and healing practices since time immemorial. Treaties 8 and 11 were signed in 1899 and 1921–22 within a vision of peace and coexistence between Indigenous Peoples and newcomers to the territories. Chief Monfwi, signing Treaty 11 in Fort Rae (now Behchokǫ̀), said, "As long as the sun rises, the river flows, and the land does not move, we will not be restricted from our way of life."[3] At the time, treatymakers for Indigenous Nations in what is now the Northwest Territories asked for medicine and doctors for their people, but the treaty commissioners explained that it would be impossible to deliver medical care across such a vast territory. At the same time, they assured the people that "the Government would always be ready to avail itself of any opportunity of affording medical service."[4]

The treaties did not clarify in writing any federal government responsibility to provide medicine or health care, even though it was understood by Indigenous signatories to be included in the terms of the treaties.[5] Inuit, including Inuvialuit, did not sign historical treaties, but a vision for improving the well-being of Inuit was key to the vision of modern treaties that led to the creation of Nunavut and the Inuvialuit Settlement Region. Indigenous Peoples understood treaty with newcomers to their lands as creating enduring relationships within which future generations could flourish.[6]

Instead, and unfortunately, health care has been dismissed by the federal government as outside of the treaty relationship. It was the arrival of newcomers and establishment of settler communities that expanded Western medicine and health infrastructure, first through churches and church hospitals, sometimes by travelling doctors, and then by federal and territorial governments. Newcomers brought diseases with them or created new environmental risks that damaged the land and made people sick.[7] As Florence Barnaby shares in this volume: "Our community is hit hard with cancer. We now have cancer screening in place for residents every two years. We blame it on the pollution coming downstream from the South into the Mackenzie River."

Historian Liza Piper writes about how health care was provided in the North at first for the newcomers to the territory rather than for Indigenous Peoples. This was the case up until the 1940s and 1950s, when the creation of medical and public health infrastructure in the North established an uneven geography of medical care and a structure of indifference that continues today.[8] The expansion of the medical system has continued to benefit non-Indigenous people working at mines and in government roles, while Indigenous health care has been framed as an act of compassion predicated on racist attitudes[9] and tied to a broader project of assimilation.[10] This unevenness of health care in the North has also meant that Indigenous Peoples must travel for health care. Since the arrival of Western medicine, Indigenous Peoples have been required to leave their home territories to access medical care, while the burgeoning use of aviation enabled "mercy flights" in emergency situations between Northern locales and Southern hospitals.[11]

When tuberculosis (TB) became epidemic in Northern Indigenous communities in the mid-twentieth century, rather than improving Northern hospitals, the federal government sent Northerners to hospitals in the South for treatment.[12] By 1960 there were twenty-two "Indian hospitals," all in Southern Canada, with the Camsell Hospital in Edmonton being the largest.[13] These hospitals treated patients from across a vast Northern geography within a vision of medical care that was racially segregated (in that the hospitals were only for Indigenous Peoples), inferior (as the quality of care was less and included experimentation on patients), and assimilative (as the hospitals removed peoples from their land, language, and way of life and encouraged assimilation into mainstream Canadian society).[14] This established a pattern whereby health care was centred in Southern cities instead of in Northern communities.

Today, health care in the territory is delivered by the Northwest Territories Health and Social Services Authority (NTHSSA), the Hay River Health and Social Services Authority (HRHSSA), the Tłı̨chǫ Community Services Agency (TCSA), and the Department of Health and Social Services (DHSS). Services are concentrated in the regional centres of Yellowknife, Inuvik, and Hay River — all of which have hospitals. Smaller communities have a health centre that may be staffed with a nurse or paramedic along with community health representatives. As well, doctors and mobile clinics travel to smaller communities.

As you will read in the narratives that follow, to access some specialist services and treatments, patients travel to Yellowknife or to Southern hospitals. This geography of care is a legacy of how health care came to the territory and the patterns of health infrastructure and medical travel that were established. This is another way of seeing structural racism in practice: if Indigenous lives in small communities mattered, there would be better health care services and infrastructure provided locally. The often-told story shared by Indigenous Northerners makes the structure of indifference visible: an Indigenous person in a small community goes to the local nursing station again and again, given only Tylenol for what ails them, only to find out later they have advanced cancer or another life-threatening disease. This is what happened to Clara Bates and others in her community, as she tells in her story in this volume. Others have had a similar experiences, like Délı̨nę Elder Morris Neyelle: "After several years seeking treatment for ongoing stomach pain, Morris flew himself to Yellowknife ... [He] was immediately diagnosed with late-stage colon cancer, undergoing surgery the next day. He passed away within weeks."[15]

There is still much work to be done to improve medical care in the North. At a time of crisis, no one should have to deal with administrative barriers to getting the care they need, and no one should have to be alone when they receive the worst news of their life. Yet this is happening to the many Northern residents who are forced to leave their family and travel down South to receive a cancer diagnosis in a city and within a health care system that many don't know how to navigate on their own.

Locum[16] doctors without knowledge of the unique needs of Northerners temporarily come to the North to gain experience and practise on patients. The requirements for cultural awareness are often left to the wayside. This is cause for concern from a human rights perspective and because many patients may not be receiving the proper care they deserve. People are often dismissed without the care of a culturally informed medical professional.

Public health care in what is now Canada has allowed many to thrive and live long lives. But for Indigenous Peoples the benefit has been questionable, and in Dene, Métis, and Inuit territories in the North, health inequities have been long lasting and persistent. Health care is thus "a terrain of racism and colonialism ... that costs lives."[17]

The Social Determinants of Cancer in the North

About 111 cases of cancer are diagnosed each year in the Northwest Territories, with lung, colorectal, breast, and prostate cancers being the most commonly detected.[18] There are screening programs here for colorectal, breast, and cervical cancers.[19] But some contributors to this book wonder if there was cancer in the North in the past: "Did we have cancer before there was sugar in our communities? I don't know," shares Ruth Wright. Another contributor says that she heard stories from older generations who knew about cancer and witnessed people who went from healthy to skin and bones. Back then there were no nurses or doctors, so the people did what they could to make them comfortable. In a podcast, contributor Lianne Mantla-Look shared that there is no word for cancer in the Tłı̨chǫ language; instead, it is usually translated as "strong disease."[20]

Research studies don't often include Northern Indigenous cancer patient perspectives. And not all of them consider the social determinants of health that contribute to cancer. This would root understandings of health and well-being in individual and community social contexts. For Northern Indigenous cancer patients, the ongoing colonialism, systemic racism, and spatial inequities related to the health care system's concentration in urban centres contributes to poor health and lack of well-being. But then again, strong connections to the land, language, culture, and community keep people healthy.

Many contributors to this book faced a cancer diagnosis and treatment during the COVID-19 pandemic. In Northern regions, as elsewhere, policies and programs to prevent or limit the spread of COVID-19 were developed quickly and evaluated later.[21] The pandemic policy response had a huge impact on cancer patients, who are considered immunocompromised and at risk of severe disease, and who are often required to travel for their treatment. Many patients spent months alternating between medical travel and isolation, with limited supports.

Indeed, most cancer patients in the North, at some point in their diagnosis or treatment, will travel for medical care. When a patient travels to a larger centre for services not available in their home community, this is called medical travel. Colloquially in the North, people might just say "medical," as in, "I have to go South on medical." As you will read, this can be a huge burden for Northern cancer patients, who "must travel thousands of kilometres and navigate complex and unwelcoming health care systems to be treated for cancer."[22] A trip for a single appointment can take several days.[23] People from the most remote communities experience the highest burden of medical travel, and mobility or illness related issues make any journey even more challenging.[24] Child care is not an allowable medical travel expense, and children cannot travel as a non-medical escort for their parent or caregiver. A patient with dependent family members has to deal with all of this on top of enduring the emotional and physical effects of cancer and cancer treatment. At the time of publication, the NWT medical travel policy covers return airfare, interfacility ambulance services for emergency medical evacuations, and some support for meals, accommodation, and ground transportation. In some cases, the expenses of a non-medical escort to accompany and assist the patient can be covered.[25]

Perhaps this explains the findings of one research team that patients living farther away from health care facilities experience worse health outcomes.[26] Barriers to medical travel can lead to delays in receiving care, avoidance of care seeking, poorer outcomes, and higher costs.[27] In general, the current medical travel policy framework in the Northwest Territories does not sufficiently bridge barriers to accessing care and may reinforce health inequities.[28] This includes people who must travel to give birth under the medical evacuation for birth policy.[29]

One way to improve care is to support shared decision making. Patients and their escorts can be supported and provided with information throughout their journey to receive cancer care.[30] This means sharing better information about a patient's medical travel, better communication and awareness across jurisdictions, ensuring the financial burden for patients and escorts is reduced as much as possible, and ensuring patients have access to facilitated appointments with medical escorts or cancer navigators.[31] Capacity can be built within the existing cancer care system to support Indigenous Northerners who have appointments far away from home.[32] This can mean increasing cultural safety and awareness among health care providers, facilitating respectful and patient-centred care, and expanding access to medical services in Indigenous languages.[33]

Implementing changes to help Indigenous and biomedical systems work together better can also improve the experience of patients. Sophie Roher and colleagues write about bringing Indigenous healing practices and biomedical hospital care together at Stanton Territorial Hospital through three frameworks: integration, interdependence, and revisioning relationship.[34] Nicole Redvers and colleagues share that equitable and culturally safe health care includes the integration of Indigenous medicine into the territorial health system. This would not only benefit patients, but in co-designing access to Indigenous health, all Northerners would benefit.[35] Patients should have the option to draw on their ancestral medicines as they need to and when they choose to. For example, Catherine Boucher used spruce gum, just as her grandfather taught her to. On the other hand, Elizabeth Biscaye followed the wisdom of her father that biomedical healing works best for Western diseases.

Some also call for decolonization of the health system. Decolonizing medical travel can mean redesigning and evaluating a comprehensive medical travel framework and redefining what access to health care means in collaboration between Indigenous, territorial, and federal governments.[36] Decolonizing cancer care means that there is Indigenous leadership within the system, locally contextualized goals and priorities, improved access in remote areas to services at all steps of the cancer care continuum, a reflection of Indigenous values of health, family, and community; culturally competent patient navigation and support; and the involvement of Indigenous participants in medical and health services research.[37] Another way of decolonizing health care is returning to story and to the experiences of patients: patient experiences need to be included in redesigning health systems.[37] To plan cancer services, it's important "to listen to the cancer patients about their experiences and what is important to them."[38]

Stories as Guidance

In this book, each storyteller shares in their own way, and in their own words, what their experience with cancer has been like. These stories are raw and real and human. Storytellers share about the roller coaster of emotions felt by individuals, the lasting impacts of residential schooling on families and communities, the failures of the health system, and the strength of culture and community. *Book of Hope* storytellers also share generously about the care and support provided to them throughout their diagnosis, treatment, and whatever came afterwards. This includes their experiences with nurses, doctors, and other professionals within the health care system but also with family, friends, and community members. We also hear about the role of cancer support groups and organizations like Goba Care, created by Melinda Laboucan. She has brought an ethic of community care and Dene Law into an organization that helps Northerners in Edmonton when they are there on medical travel.[40] For many, cancer has become a turning point in their lives, a moment at which everything changed.

Being able to share our stories can be a remedy in itself, and we are thankful to be a small part of the healing journey of many of the storytellers in this book. They show us that, when life borders on death, what matters is the love and support of family and friends. Bearing witness to the stories in this book has been a remarkably moving experience for us all. Survivors live life with a newfound perspective, and this reminds us to be thankful for every breath, for every waking moment, and for every person who comes and goes for they all have a teaching. Death is an inevitable part of life, yet that shouldn't stop us from living out our days to the fullest even when death knocks on our doorstep. If we can overcome the fear of living and dying, we have won at life — there is no losing.

Through their stories, these Northerners also share guidance for others like them, making this book like a cancer support group of its own. It creates a shared and safe space to support each other. This book is by and for people with cancer, but we think you'll find there's something that pretty much everyone can take from it.

All the stories in this book were compiled by Agnes Pascal, originally from Fort McPherson, Northwest Territories. She has experienced cancer herself, and so have many of her family, friends, and community members. When Agnes was diagnosed with cancer, she recognized the need for more support and resources for Northern peoples. So, she founded the Inuvik Cancer Support Group. The stories shared in that group inspired the creation of *Book of Hope*. From 2020 to 2023, Agnes reached out across the territory to gather stories from cancer survivors. Some of the contributors wrote their own stories for the book, while others were interviewed by Agnes and their story was created by the *Book of Hope* team based on a transcript of the interview. At the end of the book are advice and recommendations for key audiences for this book: medical professionals, decision makers, caregivers, and cancer patients.

Katłı̨à Lafferty and Sara Komarnisky supported Agnes in the creation of the book, as members of an editorial team. Katłı̨à Lafferty is a Northern Dene author and journalist from the Yellowknives First Nation. She has written and published Northern stories (true and based on truth) in several bestselling fiction and nonfiction works. Sara Komarnisky is a settler author, researcher, and public scholar who has lived in Yellowknife since 2018. She has researched and published on various topics about well-being, belonging, and the US and Canadian North.

The three of us have made a great team: we all have experience with medical travel from the Northwest Territories and with the survival or loss of loved ones who were diagnosed with cancer, and Katłıà and Sara have complementary experience as editors and writers. We supported each other in editing the stories, organizing them into a manuscript, and navigating the publication process.

The stories are organized around water and waterways. Water connects us all, everywhere. Water connects landscapes and communities all across the Northwest Territories. Water is important for travelling, for hunting, harvesting, and fishing, for our survival, and sometimes for our healing. As Agnes says, "Water is healing for me. I'm always drawn to the river when I need clarity and grounding."

Take care of yourself while reading these stories. They are about what it's really like to have cancer in the North, including all the parts that are really, really hard. Contributors also share about their lives and about things that they and others have experienced — residential schooling, being sent to an Indian hospital, addiction, mental health challenges, the deaths of friends and family members. Alongside the hard stuff, there is a lot of hope in these pages.

If you find yourself struggling, put the book down for a while and find someone to talk to. Those who have personal, family, or intergenerational experiences of residential school can call the National Residential School Crisis Line at 1-866-925-4419. Help is available in the NWT at #811.

Notes

1. Government of the Northwest Territories (1998) Official Languages Act. https://www.justice.gov.nt.ca/en/files/legislation/official-languages/official-languages.a.pdf.
2. Rene M.J. Lamothe (1996), "It Was Only a Treaty": Treaty 11 According to the Dene of the Mackenzie Valley. Ottawa: Royal Commission on Aboriginal Peoples, 14-15.
3. Tłıchǫ Government (n.d.) Chronology of the Tłıchǫ Negotiation Process. Available at: https://www.tlicho.ca/cec-assembly/our-story/chronology.
4. Dennis F.K. Madill (1986) *Treaty Research Report - Treaty Eight (1899)*, Treaties and Historical Research Centre, Indian and Northern Affairs Canada, https://www.rcaanc-cirnac.gc.ca/eng/1100100028809/1564415096517.
5. Crystal Milligan, Stephanie Irlbacher-Fox, and Mark J. Dobrow (2023) "Strengthening Policy for First Nations Self-Determination in Health: An Analysis of Problems, Politics, and Policy Related to Medical Travel in Northwest Territories," *Health Reform Observer* 10, 3. Also see Rene Fumoleau (1973) *As Long as This Land Shall Last: A History of Treaty 8 and Treaty 11, 1870-1939*, University of Calgary Press; Aimée Craft and Alice Lebihan (2021) *The Treaty Right to Health: A Sacred Obligation*, National Collaborating Centre for Indigenous Health.
6. Gina Starblanket and Dallas Hunt (2020) *Covid-19, the Numbered Treaties, and the Politics of Life*, Yellowhead Institute.

7   Liza Piper (2023) *When Disease Came to this Country: Epidemics and Colonialism in Northern North America*, Cambridge University Press; John Sandlos and Arn Keeling (2016) "Toxic Legacies, Slow Violence, and Environmental Injustice at Giant Mine, Northwest Territories," *The Northern Review* 42.
8   Piper, *When Disease Came to this Country*; Mary Jane McCallum and Adele Perry (2018) *Structures of Indifference: An Indigenous Life and Death in a Canadian City*, University of Manitoba Press.
9   Liza Piper (2021) "Diphtheria Antitoxin and Tales of Mercy in Northern Health Care," *Canadian Bulletin of Medical History* 38(2).
10 Mary Jane McCallum (2005) "This Last Frontier: Isolation and Aboriginal Health," *Canadian Bulletin of Medical History* 22(1).
11 Piper, "Diphtheria Antitoxin and Tales of Mercy."
12 Milligan et.al. "Strengthening Policy," 5.
13 Maureen Lux (2016) *Separate Beds: A History of Indian Hospitals in Canada, 1920s-1980s*, University of Toronto Press.
14 Lux, *Separate Beds*; Laurie Meijer Drees (2013) *Healing Histories: Stories from Canada's Indian Hospitals*, University of Alberta Press; Sara Komarnisky, Paul Hackett, Sylvia Abonyi, and Courtney Heffernan (2015), "'Years Ago': Reconciliation and First Nations Narratives of Tuberculosis in the Canadian Prairie Provinces," *Critical Public Health*, 26(4).
15 Stephanie Irlbacher-Fox (2022) "In Memoriam, Elder Morris Neyelle, Délı̨nę," *Xàgots'eèhk'ǫ̀ Journal* 1(1): 158–159.
16 A locum is a travelling doctor who fills the place of a colleague or an empty position. In the Northwest Territories, locum doctors take on patients temporarily, coming North to work for a period of time and then returning home.
17 McCallum and Perry, *Structures of Indifference*, 134.
18 GNWT Department of Health and Social Services (n.d.) "Cancer in the NWT," https://www.cancernwt.ca/services/what-cancer/cancer-nwt; GNWT Department of Health and Social Services (2014) "Cancer in the Northwest Territories 2001-2010, Fact Sheet 1-12," https://www.hss.gov.nt.ca/sites/hss/files/nwt-cancer-fact-sheets.pdf; T. Kue Young, Janet J. Kelly, Jeppe Friborg, Leena Soinen, and Kai O. Wong (2016) "Cancer among Circumpolar Populations: An Emerging Public Health Concern," *International Journal of Circumpolar Health* 75(1).
19 NWT Health and Social Services Authority (n.d.) "Cancer Screening Programs," https://www.nthssa.ca/en/services/cancer-screening-programs.
20 Lianne Mantla-Look and Dr. Patricia Strachan (2024) "Indigenous and Northern Lens on Communication in Serious Illness," podcast, *Radical Nurse Talk*, https://radicalnursetalk.podbean.com/e/indigenous-and-northern-lens-on-communication-in-serious-illness/
21 Katherine Fleury and Susan Chatwood (2023) "Canadian Northern and Indigenous Health Policy Responses to the First Wave of COVID-19," *Scandanavian Journal of Public Health* 51.
22 Janet Jull, Amanda J. Sheppard, Alex Hizaka, Inuit Medical Interpreter Team, Gwen Barton, Paula Doering, Danielle Dorshner, Nancy Edgecombe, Megan Ellis, Ian D. Graham, Mara Habash, Gabrielle Jodouin, Lynn Kilabuk, Theresa Koonoo, Carolyn Robers, and Mamisarvik Healing Centre Team (2021) "Experience of Inuit in Canada who Travel from Remote Settings for Cancer Care and Impacts on Decision Making," *BMC Health Services Research* 21(328).
23 Milligan et.al. "Strengthening Policy."

24 Kate Kerber, Fariba Kolahdooz, Meeka Otway, Melinda Laboucan, Se Lim Jang, Sue Lawrence, Suzanne Aronyk, Matthew Quinn, Stephanie Irlbacher-Fox, Crystal Milligan, Sabrina Broadhead, Debbie DeLancey, Andre Corriveau, Sangita Sharma (2019) "Opportunities for Improving Patient Experiences among Medical Travellers from Canada's Far North: A Mixed-Methods Study," *BMJ Open Access*, 9.

25 Government of the Northwest Territories (2015) "49.06 Medical Travel," policy document, https://www.eia.gov.nt.ca/sites/eia/files/content/49.06-medical-travel-revised.pdf.

26 Charlotte Kelly, Claire Hulme, Tracey Farragher, and Graham Clarke (2016) "Are Differences in Travel Time or Distance to Healthcare for Adults in Global North Countries Associated with an Impact on Health Outcomes? A Systematic Review," *BMJ Open Access* 6(11).

27 Kerber et.al, "Opportunities for improving patient experiences," 7.

28 Milligan et.al. "Strengthening Policy," 14.

29 Pertice M. Moffitt and Ardene Robinson Vollman (2006) "At What Cost to Health? Tlicho Women's Medical Travel for Childbirth," *Contemporary Nurse* 22.

30 Kerber et.al, "Opportunities for Improving Patient Experiences,"; Jull et.al., "Experience of Inuit."

31 Kerber et.al, "Opportunities for Improving Patient Experiences." This study also advocates for better communication between healthcare providers: T. Kue Young, Janet J. Kelly, Jeppe Friborg, Leena Soinen, and Kai O. Wong (2016) "Cancer among Circumpolar Populations: An Emerging Public Health Concern," *International Journal of Circumpolar Health* 75(1).

32 Jull et.al., "Experience of Inuit."

33 Kerber et.al, "Opportunities for Improving Patient Experiences."

34 Sophie Isabelle Grace Roher, Paul Andrew, Susan Chatwood, Kimberly Fairman, Tracey Galloway, Angela Mashford-Pringle, and Jennifer L. Gibson (2023) "Envisioning Indigenous and Biomedical Healthcare Collaboration at Stanton Territorial Hospital, Northwest Territories," *International Journal of Circumpolar Health*, 82.

35 Nicole Redvers, Justina Marianayagam, and Be'sha Blondin (2019) "Improving access to Indigenous medicine for patients in hospital-based settings: a challenge for health systems in northern Canada," *International Journal of Circumpolar Health* 78.

36 Milligan et.al. "Strengthening Policy."

37 Matthew Beckett, Katherine Cole, Mitchell White, Jessica Chan, Jason McVicar, Danielle Rodin, Mark Clemons, Jean-Marc Bourque (2021) "Decolonizing Cancer Care in Canada," *Journal of Cancer Policy* 30.

38 Rhiannon Cooper, Nathaniel J. Pollock, Zander Affleck, Laura Bain, Nanna Lund Hansen, Kelsey Robertson, and Susan Chatwood (2021) "Patient healthcare experiences in the Northwest Territories, Canada: An Analysis of News Media Articles," *International Journal of Circumpolar Health* 80(1).

39 Ruth A. Robertson (2001) "Living with a Diagnosis of Cancer in Canada's Western Arctic," MA Thesis, Royal Roads University.

40 Goba Care was founded by Melinda Laboucan. It is a non-profit that supports Northwest Territories and Nunavut residents who have to travel to Edmonton for medical appointments. Goba offers multifaceted support — everything from connecting to services, helping understand the medical system, to organizing beading circles, and creating care packages for those who are sick or welcoming a new baby.

Annie Firth-Jones

HAY RIVER

I'm originally from Fort McPherson. I'm Gwich'in. I'm also a two-time cancer survivor. My mom is Mary Firth senior and my dad was William Firth. My dad's first marriage was to Mary Sibbeston, and she was from Hay River. So that was my connection with Hay River. I went there to go to school and I also met all the Sibbestons. I had ten brothers, four step-brothers, one step-sister, and one adopted sister. I've lived in Hay River for the past thirty years.

Most of my siblings went to residential school in Hay River and the rest of them went to Grollier Hall in Inuvik. Me, my dad wouldn't let me go. I went to school in Fort McPherson until grade 7, then I did correspondence, then I went to college in Edmonton. The college was a residential school, but it wasn't acknowledged as a residential school in terms of the residential school settlement.[1]

When I look back now, I realize I blocked some things that happened from my memory. When I heard that they found the children in Kamloops,[2] my son found me thrashing and crying in my bed. My son couldn't calm me down. He called the ambulance and I was taken to the hospital. I explained that I had a dream, and the doctor asked me to share it with her.

I dreamt I was standing on the shoreline and my dad was holding on to my hand. We could see a boat coming. I tried to get away. The boat came and a person came out in dark black clothes and nuns followed. I tried to get away. Not far from me there were women and children crying.

I also told my sister about my dream. She said that was exactly how she was taken away on the boat when she went to residential school. I still don't really understand it. Part of her history was with me, so it wasn't a dream.

After that dream I started remembering things that happened to me. I couldn't work and I had a hard time sleeping. I could hear crying. I talked to a counsellor and saw a psychologist and was told I needed trauma counselling. So, one spring, I went to a trauma centre. The first thing they do is take everything away from you. No phone, no TV, no radio — nothing for six weeks, and that was the best thing that ever happened to me. All the staff were Indigenous.

When I graduated from the social work program in Fort Smith, I went to Yellowknife to do my practicum for a month when my supervisor called me and said, "Inuvik wants you because they are short staffed and you are Gwich'in; you know the people, you know the history." So, I went to Inuvik and started working but I wasn't feeling good. I went to the doctor, and they did all these tests but there was nothing showing up. Then I really got sick, so I went to the doctor in Inuvik, and they sent me out of the community the next day to do tests for cancer.

My first diagnosis was stage three colon cancer. I received the diagnosis on 9/11, the morning the twin towers came down. My consultation called for immediate surgery, chemo, and radiation. The treatment was brutal: most of my treatment was in Edmonton. I had chemotherapy and radiation for four months in Edmonton, and further chemotherapy treatment in Yellowknife.

In Edmonton, I took the shuttle to my appointments; it picked me up every day. My husband helped take care of me. He got me up every day. But one day as I lay on the couch I told my husband to tell the shuttle driver to go on without me because I wasn't going back. He said, "Okay." After that, I don't know how long I was lying there. I looked at the glow around my phone and I thought, "Who am I to give up when all those people are calling me and praying for me?" So, I got up and said to my husband, "Let's go." The shuttle driver was still waiting for me. That's the day I decided to live.

Six years later I was working on the reserve in Hay River as a counsellor.[3] Public health workers came in one morning and said they had to do a TB test on me because one of my clients tested positive. That's how I found out I had cancer again. I also had a cough that I couldn't get rid of. I didn't feel like it was a cold. The doctor said, "Let's just do an x-ray," and when he called me back, he told me I had lung cancer. The first question he asked was, "Do you smoke? How long have you smoked?" I said, "I never smoked." When I was growing up my dad was always smoking his long pipe and I would sit as close to him as I could because I liked the smell of the tobacco, and the doctor said, "That's the worst kind of smoke."

Again, I had to go to Edmonton and have surgery. I was at the hospital early in the morning, the first patient in the surgery room. When I woke up after surgery, I felt good. I thought, "I'm going to have things in my control now." After I spoke to my doctor that day, I made up my mind. I discharged myself. My husband came and I said, "Get me my clothes. I feel good and I want to go." My husband was not in agreement with my decision. But I was determined. He got my clothes together but the nurses said, "You can't leave, you need to take the IV out." I said, "If you don't take it out, I'll take it out myself." They called the doctor and he said, "No you can't leave," but I said, "I'm going." So, I did. I left.

I walked outside, and saw someone I knew, and they said, "I thought you were going for surgery?" I said, "I had my surgery." He said, "When?" I said, "this morning." Then he said, "Turn around and get back there." He was mad at me. I said, "No. Just leave me alone. Let me be." I went back to Hay River, and a month later the doctor called me to talk about treatment. I said, "I'm not taking chemo. What else can you offer me?" After long conversations, the doctor and I agreed that I would take chemotherapy in pill form rather than liquid form. This meant the treatment period would be twice as long for me. Due to my contact with an individual who tested positive for tuberculosis, I was also placed on medication for TB for a year. There were times I felt sick and worn out, but I was determined to beat this disease. I made a deal with the cancer. I told the cancer, "You do your part, and I'll do mine." I kept praying and thought of the many people suffering and I thought, "Who am I to give in?"

When I took my last pill, I was sitting at my computer at work. I thought, "I'm in my seventies, what am I still doing at work?" So, I resigned right then and there. My mom was dying that year, too. She phoned me and asked me to come home and look after her. She wanted to die at home. I went.

After my first cancer diagnosis, I was in a program called Cancer Connection[4] for about eight years. It really helped me. It was a very supportive program. They paired me with other people around the same age as me with the same type of cancer. One time a man said, "I'm terminal. It's just me and my wife. I don't have much time. I insist that my wife keep working. Every morning, I get up and I pray to be here until she comes to have coffee with me. Then I pray that I can have a little bit of soup by lunch." I talked to him for about two or three months. Then one day I got a call and was told that he was gone. I said, "I hope he died peacefully." He had died in his sleep. Another person I met through Cancer Connection told me, "I'm so glad I have you to talk with and to listen to me. I don't want my family to know how bad I'm feeling." Someone else said, "Thank you for listening."

My husband died of dementia. I looked after him for two years. He was always very supportive. He would do everything for me when I had cancer. Sometimes I would feel sorry for him because I would say, "I'm so hungry." Then he would make me a can of soup, but I would suddenly lose my appetite and not want it anymore. But he said it was okay; it was the thought that counted. My husband's support system was his lifelong friend circle and his sisters. I always had a good support system, especially in my husband. One time I was listening to him talking to someone and they asked him, "What did you learn from Anne?" And he said, "Patience. I learned patience." I think that's what most caregivers would say. You want to do more; you want to fix it, but there comes a time when you have to realize that you can't fix it. Just being there is enough. Sometimes people don't want to talk.

I was angry when I found out I had cancer. I asked, "Why me?" Especially the second diagnosis. I was angry because I never smoked. I had quit drinking and was on a healthy path and I still got sick. But cancer taught me a lot about self-awareness. About taking things one day at a time. About realizing that all we have is right now.

I went to the Cross Cancer for my treatment, and it was beautiful and comforting. Even though it's not a place where anyone wants to be, at least people are together; there's comfort in being together. During my first few sessions I was not looking happy, and this person said, "I know sitting there waiting seems like a long time but please don't ever miss an appointment. There are many people just wanting to get in for an appointment and we are lucky." That really opened my eyes.

Sometimes people think I'm strong, but I get annoyed because I don't want to be strong. I don't want my kids to know how bad I'm feeling. Sometimes people say, "I feel for you and I wish I could take your pain." I used to feel scared when a follow-up appointment was coming up. Your imagination can play tricks on you. Right now, I'm waiting on test results. I had to go to the dentist, which is something I don't like to do. They took x-rays, whispered to one another and then took another x-ray. The dentist told me I have a growth in my jaw and sent me to see a specialist, so I'm waiting to see the specialist. I've had three colonoscopies in the past three months. They have found polyps. I'm still waiting for results.

Growing up, my family always went to church: morning, afternoon, and evening service. Except for my dad; he never went to church. I always wondered if there really was a God. When things went wrong, I would think, "How could God do this?" It just puzzled me. But before my mom died, she wanted me to be with her. One night she asked me to call the nurses and said, "Anne I think this is it." We were holding hands, my mom was smiling, and she said "They're singing. They're singing. Don't you hear it?" I saw a little feather that dissolved after she took her last breath. That was her spirit. I was so amazed. She looked so at peace. All her wrinkles were gone. I was happy for her and I was happy for myself. That was a gift she gave me. I now believed.

One morning when I was in treatment, our group was standing up and holding hands and sharing how we felt that day. One man there always came to help me. He said, "I got something for you." I said, "What is it?" He handed me a little flower and said, "This is the first flower I saw this spring," It was a buttercup. As he gave it to me, a feather fell down. I put it in my bible, and I thought, "Oh, my mom's with me." I had to look at my spirituality. I came to the conclusion that I was afraid to believe. But believing is magnificence. There is power when you believe. There are always signs.

If you are first learning that you have been diagnosed with cancer, put your feet down and get grounded. Take some deep breaths and sit with it. You don't have to say anything. You'll take one step at a time and know that I'm here and others will be too. When you are ready, reach out. People want to help. If you are wondering about something and not feeling good, tell someone. Take one step at a time and know that people will be there for you, and they do want to help.

Notes

1. Residential school survivors took the government to court and won, and the result was an Indian Residential Schools Settlement Agreement to address the legacy of the schools. The agreement included payment for all eligible former students, a process to assess and compensate claims for sexual or physical abuse, measures to support healing, commemorative activities, and the establishment of a Truth and Reconciliation Commission.
2. In May 2021, Tk'emlúps te Secwépemc announced the finding of the remains of 215 children who were buried on the grounds of the former Kamloops Indian Residential School. This finding led to a national outpouring of grief and outrage.
3. Kátł'odeeche First Nation Reserve, also sometimes called Hay River Reserve.
4. Cancer Connection is an online resource from the Canadian Cancer Society: www.cancerconnection.ca.

Kelsey Townend (McGinley)

HAY RIVER

I have lived in Hay River for nearly half my life. I am raising my three beautiful sons with my husband in the North. I love the people here and admire the way everyone cares for one another. Even a small community like Hay River can come together and support each other through the toughest of times. I am incredibly grateful my life led me here.

When I catch myself not smiling or laughing less, when feelings of depression and anxiety creep up on me, when I begin to question my life and its purpose, or when I get lonely and angry, I remember it's coming up to the day I was diagnosed with cancer, and it all makes sense. In February 2016, I was diagnosed with stage two choriocarcinoma at 30 years old. At that time, I was a mother of two young boys. I was forced to leave my home and my children. I had to leave everything behind and travel to Edmonton for four months where I had chemotherapy three times a week, for up to eight hours a day in a chair, in an otherwise empty room at the Cross Cancer Institute. It felt incredibly heavy and terrifying.

I shaved my head before my hair started to fall out — an attempt to keep something within my control. I was so sick at times that I wasn't able to lift my head up. I remember throwing up often and aggressively. I would have massive nosebleeds at the same time. My mother was my main caretaker. She would sit or stand near me to make sure I didn't collapse. I would usually just be in my underwear and a tank top due to the dramatic changes in feeling hot or cold. I can't imagine, as a mother, having to watch my child suffer so immensely. Without my mom, I would not have survived.

I had an aggressive cancer that required an aggressive treatment, which meant I had to have an extensive amount of chemotherapy treatments administered to give me the best chance of surviving. I remember wondering, "What kind of survival is this?" I was away from my home, and I would only see my children briefly once a month and then I would have to return to the Cross Cancer Institute for more treatment. Being separated from my boys was the most difficult part of the experience.

I came close to dying on many occasions. During chemotherapy, I also struggled with various infections because I was completely depleted and my immune system was compromised.

What no one warned me about is navigating life after surviving cancer. Somehow, I thought that after surviving cancer, life would return back to normal. I thought I could go back home and pick up where I left off. That was not the case, and it was a huge disappointment. I felt as if a large part of who I was before I got cancer was gone, and it was. I felt disconnected from my children, I didn't feel beautiful, my skin was different, my body was different, and even my memory was failing me.

I was later diagnosed with avascular necrosis in both my humeral heads (shoulders), which required shoulder replacements post treatment. My left shoulder was replaced in 2020 and my right shoulder in 2023. I continue to struggle with self-image, depression, anxiety, post-traumatic stress disorder, chronic pain, and other things.

I believe I died for four months and somehow made it out alive. I survived, and because I survived, I thought I didn't have the right to be angry, sad, anxious or depressed. I thought to myself, "I should be making the most out of every single moment." I would love to say I do, but I still struggle to navigate surviving. A lot of days I feel broken. I'm surrounded by so many people, but still, I feel lonely. I long for the woman I used to be, the woman I used to love and adore. I was fun, I smiled, and I laughed more. I shined a light so brightly, even in the darkest of rooms. I miss her. I lost a part of myself in those four months, and I struggle with that grief, but how can I express that when some people don't survive? At times I feel ungrateful. Survivors' guilt is real: I survived, but I don't live my life as if I survived. I question everything.

People tell me how strong they believe I am to have fought and endured chemotherapy for four months under extreme circumstances, but I don't consider myself strong or brave. I only did what I was told and hoped that I could one day get back home to my kids, no matter what that looked like.

Although I struggle with certain aspects of my life, I remind myself that I am still alive and to be thankful for that. I get to go to sleep and hopefully open my eyes to another day. I have hope. I'm not hopeful from a place of strength or courage, but from a place of fear. I fear if I don't have hope, I will lose myself completely.

Cancer does not end after a successful treatment plan. It follows you for the rest of your life. It can creep back in and remind you that you could not be here today. That reminder is a blessing and a curse.

I want to heal. I want to feel connected. I want to feel like myself again. I'm still searching and won't ever stop.

Cancer survivors, I see you, I feel you, and I understand you. There is an unspoken bond between those who have come close to death. We know that surviving can carry a certain heaviness, something you can't quite articulate, but when I meet another survivor, I feel it without saying a word. That is why I founded and solely facilitate a cancer sharing circle in Hay River, Northwest Territories, called The Karuna Group, which offers peer support to anyone affected by cancer. I care deeply for every single person who has ever attended the support group. They have become like family. A group member once said to me, "It's the coolest group of people that no one actually wants to be a part of." It always makes me laugh, because it's true. I am thankful for every one of the people who have given The Karuna Group Cancer Sharing Circle a chance. I am honoured to facilitate this group.

When I was diagnosed with cancer, it was the beginning of what would be the most challenging experience of my life. I am thankful to be in this community that cares so deeply and to have a family that loves and supports me the way they do. My family, they are my reason to never give up. They want me to thrive. I will continue to share my experiences in hope that my experiences will help someone else who may be facing a similar situation. I hope that my story may help, even if it's only for one other person to feel supported and less alone.

Catherine Boucher

FORT RESOLUTION

My family is originally from Taltson River, where the community of Rocher River was before we were relocated to Fort Resolution in the 1960s.[1] My grandfather Boniface Boucher Jr. raised me. I was about 4 years old when I was taken to residential school and went back and forth between Rocher River and residential school for most of my childhood.

I have been through a lot, but I never thought I was going to get cancer. I had just gone in for a check-up like you do when you get older. In October 2003 I was told I had cancer, the kind of cancer that only about one in a million get. I couldn't believe it. I didn't want to tell my brothers or sisters because I didn't want them to worry about me. I told my husband, Leandre, but I did not tell the kids. I didn't want everyone coming around me. I wanted to try and beat it myself on my own first.

When I was diagnosed, I could hear my grandfather whispering in my ear, "ʔ seyëz dechëndze t'ąnet'į." which in my language means, "My child, use spruce gum," and that is what I did. When I was young and travelling with my grandfather on the land I would eat spruce gum. We used to portage here and there in a little canoe travelling on Great Slave Lake and up to Taltson River. We would go up to the lake and look for ducks, any kind of wildlife you eat. Every time we stopped on the shore there would be spruce trees, and he'd take a piece and tell me, "ʔ seyëz dechëndze t'ąnet'į."

When I was told I had cancer I thought right away that I was going to use gum, spruce gum. So that's what I did. In the beginning, I tried mixing it with juniper. I experimented. I wanted to see how it worked and try it on myself. You get it from spruce trees, or from tamarack, any of the evergreen trees you can find. I didn't want to boil it, because I thought if I boiled it and drank the liquid, I'd have to go to the bathroom too fast. I wanted it to stay in my body longer. If I eat it, it'll go in my body and eventually go into the blood system and travel to wherever it needed to go to do the work. I crushed my gum to look like salt or sugar, I kept it in the fridge, and I ate a tablespoon of crushed spruce gum every twelve hours.

The doctors wanted to set a date to give me a hysterectomy in November 2003. I didn't tell my doctor that I was using spruce gum until then. I told her I didn't want to get a hysterectomy right away, so from October to January they agreed to monitor me and then take a look again. My cancer was rare; it was kind of a liquid and the size of a loonie. I started eating that spruce gum in August and I just kept eating and eating it. In January, they called me up to Yellowknife to look at the cancer using an ultrasound. It had shrunk. So, I said, "Well, I don't want that operation then, I'll hang on to this. I'll use my gum until it goes away or whatever." And it kept going away. They monitored me every four months. And during that entire time, I kept getting gum and crushing it and eating it like I described. I kept getting monitored and I kept eating the gum, and after about five years they told me there was no sign of cancer anymore. My doctor kept asking me what she had given me to take, but she hadn't given me anything. I guess she forgot and thought she had prescribed me medication.

Now, I encourage anyone to use spruce gum if they are sick. But you have to go out and get it yourself. You're the one who has to pray to God and tell him what you're going to use it for: to help you heal. Elders used to say that when you go in the bush you pray and then you take your medicine and then you pay the land. That's the way my grandfather used to do it. So, I did it that way, too. I notice some people on the highway now and then, just chopping on spruce trees. So, I know they're picking gum, and that is good. There's lots, we might as well take as much as we can every year. It keeps leaking out. The more you take, the more you get. The more it'll come out; it'll be in big chunks. We got to start using our natural herbs. We've got lots up here. Eventually, maybe when all this sickness goes away, I will go to more places and meet people and discuss the traditional medicines again. I want to keep promoting it. I don't mind helping, I don't mind sharing. If people want to use it, they'll use it. And I just encourage people just to try it and go out and pray and do what you have to do for yourself first. After that it'll work, I know, if you do that.

Sometimes you have that feeling, you know, when you got something bad, but you know it is going to be all right. You feel it in your heart, and you know it's real. That's the way I felt. You have got to feel positive. You have to work on yourself and be strong and think positive. That's the only way you can beat it. If you feel sad, you've got to live life!

Note

1   Rocher River was located where the Taltson River drains into Great Slave Lake, north and east of Fort Resolution. Dene have lived there since long ago, and the first cabins in the community were built by a trading chief. The community was abandoned in the late 1960s after the school burned down and the government chose not to rebuild it.

James (Jim) Lynn

DETTAH

My official name is James but I go by Jim. I was born on March 30, 1938, in Lethbridge, and I was raised there, too. I was ordained a priest on June 1, 1963. I lived most of my early life in southern Alberta. I moved North in 1986. I've been here ever since. I spent a couple months in Fort Smith but have lived in Yellowknife and Dettah ever since.

My cancer was in the esophagus. It was over twenty years ago; I almost don't remember now. I lost all my hair. They were trying to give me an intravenous injection for medicine, and it took four or five people to find a vein. The chemotherapy never bothered me. I would sit in the chair and go to work after. It never phased me or changed my lifestyle whatsoever. I've been blessed in that regard. Cancer never set me back at all, in all honesty.

The community was with me in prayer. I took my radiation in Calgary rather than Edmonton because I had a brother there. I was weak at that time, but I've been cancer free for the last twenty years or so now. I'm 85 years of age and in good health. I was in the 55+ summer games in Kamloops and won two silver medals in cycling. I still try to cycle 15 km a day. That's my life and I'm sticking to it.

I found out about the cancer because I had a lump on my chest. I was curious about it, so I went to the doctors and they diagnosed me with cancer. It's hard to say where I got it from. I used a lot of chemicals while farming when I was young, so I think I may have picked up the cancer that way. But I have no evidence of that. There's no cancer history in our family other than my brother, who died of throat cancer.

Cancer is not something that scared or frightened me. It was just another crisis, difficulty, or trial that the Lord sent to me. When He sends trials, he sends strengths and blessings to deal with the trials. I've always believed that thy will be done, not my will, not my wishes, but thy will. It's not a question of getting down on my knees and begging God to live but saying, "It's in your hands, Lord. I trust that I've had the time and space in this world, and I trust I've done what you've asked of me to the best of my ability." It didn't make me give up on life. I continued the journey and made the most of the situation I found myself in. I told my family, and they were concerned and wondered how long I'd be around for. But when they realized that the treatment was working, they started to relax a bit.

I was a parish priest, but after a couple of years in community I met my wife, an Indigenous lady. I chose to get married, so I left the active priesthood and started a family. I got permission from Rome, and the bishops recognize my great love of the Lord, so they allowed me to continue in the ministry. I'm chaplain at the jail. I joke that I've got a life sentence — I've been there for twenty years. I'm also chaplain in the community of Dettah, where I've lived for the past twenty-five years. I go to the jail and the bishop's office every day.

I have three daughters. and a great love of Elvis and his music. When I was sick, I remember my youngest daughter saying, "Dad, I don't want you to leave but if you do, you're going to meet your friend Elvis." It was so beautiful.

I just love the sacred scriptures. If someone tells me their story, I go to the scriptures, New and Old Testament, to give them strength. I often go to the first book of Joshua and share the message to be strong and courageous, to walk with the world, and to leave it in God's hands. That is the message I want to share with anyone who has cancer. Jesus doesn't abandon you when you have cancer. He's with you throughout it and He'll support you. Just live every day that you've got. Enjoy every moment you have with the Lord and for the Lord and show that strength and courage to the people around you so that they, too, can be strong.

We just got back from a trip to Florida. I sat in the sun and soaked it up every minute I could get. I'm aware that skin cancer is a possibility but at my age I'm ready to go when He's ready to call me.

Toni Anderson

YELLOWKNIFE

My love for the North began the summer I turned 18 years old. I had been selected to participate in a two-month-long canoe trip from Fort Liard to Inuvik with a group of seven other young adults. We slept along the shores of the Deh Cho, marvelled at the beauty of the ramparts at Fort Good Hope, and received amazing hospitality from the communities along the two rivers we travelled on. Someone once told me, "you never leave the North," and for me it was true. I came back for a winter two years after that trip and finally moved to Yellowknife in 2016 with my family.

In September 2020, I moved into a five-bedroom student housing apartment in Yellowknife with my children. It was the first place that was really mine because I had been with my ex-husband since I was eighteen, and before that, I lived with my parents. I found the lump in my breast only one week after moving in.

When I was in my 20s, I worked at CIBC, and I still have many friends who work there. Every September, they fundraise for the Run for the Cure, and my Facebook feed fills up with posts reminding people to do breast self-examinations. One of those posts inspired me to do the fateful self-exam that changed the course of my life. The lump was not particularly big, and it was slightly squishy. I thought it probably wasn't cancer, but I decided to get it checked out anyway. I am so grateful to the physician I saw at that appointment. Even though she agreed it probably wasn't cancer, she referred me for diagnostic testing anyway.

I got in right away for a mammogram and ultrasound, but I rescheduled because I didn't want to miss a clinical shift. Nursing school is really intense, and students are discouraged from scheduling appointments that might conflict with clinical practice. With hindsight, I tell my friends, "Put your health before nursing school," but it's easier said than done.

I eventually went for my mammogram and ultrasound, and I left that appointment knowing something was terribly wrong. If the mammogram technologist starts taking lots of extra pictures, something is wrong. She kept going back to the radiologist, and the radiologist kept ordering more images. I was sneaking pictures with my phone whenever she left the room so I could investigate on my own after the appointment. What I saw on the screen looked like a spider or a crab, and that is what cancer looks like. At the end of the appointment, the radiologist came in and assessed me himself. He told me that it was definitely not a cyst and that he was concerned about the images. Since this was during the COVID-19 pandemic, they didn't want to send me to Edmonton because I'd have to be isolated for two weeks when I came home and I'd miss a lot of school.[1] School had become a lifeline for me — I needed to finish my degree and become a nurse so that I would be able to provide for my children as a single mom. The decision was for the surgeon in Yellowknife to do a free-hand biopsy without imaging. They tried that, and it came back as normal tissue, but the doctor said, "That still doesn't explain it. You're going to have to go to Edmonton."

I was really worried about missing school at that point, but I went to Edmonton to do my biopsy. I was in Edmonton for one night, and then I flew back to Yellowknife. Then I was in isolation for two weeks without my kids. During that time, they stayed with their father. One day, plans were made for my kids to see me through a glass window, but my three-year-old didn't understand, and he wept over not being allowed to come into the apartment and see me. That's when my mental health began to decline. I was alone in my apartment, obsessing over the radiologist's report and the photos I'd taken of the images of the mammogram. Everything in the report indicated cancer. I knew I had cancer, just no one had told me yet.

My surgeon scheduled a follow-up appointment that was "conveniently" exactly an hour after my two-week isolation ended. The physician told me the biopsy had come back positive for cancer. The reports were dated ten days earlier. I could have been told a whole week earlier! I am still upset that I was left in that mental limbo longer than necessary.

The cancer was triple positive, which means it was estrogen, progesterone, and Her2 positive. It was grade 3, 1.9 cm in size, and did not appear to have spread to my lymph nodes, which made it clinically stage one at that point. I left in a calm state, knowing it was treatable. I knew what I was dealing with, and I knew that something could be done about it. I didn't go into a fog like people do in the movies. I remember it all very clearly.

I had a short window before I had to go back to Edmonton for an MRI.[2] I had to stay in Edmonton after my MRI because I had surgery scheduled two weeks later, and if I went back to Yellowknife, I would have had to spend the entire time home in isolation. Being away from my kids was one of the hardest parts of it all. As a student and stay-at-home mom, I was used to having my kids around me all the time. Then, suddenly, my kids were at their dad's house without me for long stretches of time. It was a devastating loss that I couldn't have my kids with me while our family was in crisis. I felt really out of control of my life.

Throughout it all, I stayed in school. I was able to attend classes remotely and ended up doing well on my exams. I was very proud of myself that I was able to complete that semester and maintain my academic success. My grades slipped a little during that semester, but not a lot. Given the circumstances, this felt like a huge accomplishment.

The results of my MRI were that my lymph nodes might be involved, so I had to have a lymph node biopsy to rule it out. It came back negative, and I went into surgery thinking I'd come out stage one. I found out two days before Christmas that there were two positive lymph nodes and that the tumour had grown from 1.9 cm to 2.5 cm during the time between my diagnostic mammogram and surgery. I was absolutely devastated about the pathology results.

I went into a very deep depression. I couldn't eat. I couldn't sleep. I was still reeling from the separation from my ex, and I was so angry that I had these irreversible changes made to my body at such a vulnerable time in my life. I was prescribed medication to sleep, which helped, but I would wake up with a jolt in the middle of the night, and I would lie in bed with my heart racing, unable to fall back asleep. I was a total mess.

One thing that was particularly hard for me as I processed my diagnosis was accepting that I needed to ask for help. I decided to ask my mom to come stay with me in Yellowknife while I underwent chemotherapy for eighteen weeks. That meant asking her to uproot her entire life, rehome her cats, find a house sitter, cancel plans, and bring only what could fit in two suitcases for the next five months. It's not easy to ask that of anyone, but my mom immediately agreed and made arrangements to come help me. She came to Yellowknife to stay with the kids when I had to leave for treatment in Edmonton and help take care of me when I came home. My best friend flew to Edmonton to be with me when I was there, so I wasn't alone. My sister travelled a few times to Edmonton to meet me during treatment as well.

When I was at the height of my depression, it was hard to imagine a happy future. I wondered if I should even bother with staying in school. I thought it would be a great waste of time away from my kids if the cancer came back. I had a lot of negative thoughts. One day, I had an epiphany: I needed to live my life as though I believed I was going to survive, even if I didn't believe it in the moment. I made all decisions based on the idea that I was going to get better, I was going to get back into full-time studies, and I was going to become a nurse. I could have sabotaged my future by making decisions based on my darkest fears, but instead, I made deliberate choices to protect my future.

The next major obstacle I faced was when I found out from the college that I'd have to move out of student housing even though I was still taking classes. Since I wasn't able to attend clinical placements, I wouldn't be able to advance to the fall semester. I would have to wait a year to join the next nursing cohort and during that time I wouldn't be a student and therefore couldn't stay in student housing. It was just too much. I called my social worker and put out a desperate post on my social media page that got picked up by the news. Aurora College eventually backed down and said I could take classes from another faculty part-time and keep my apartment. I decided to take psychology, English, and Indigenous governance. I decided to take Indigenous governance as an opportunity to learn about my own Métis heritage. It was the silver lining of my "penalty year."

During that time, I also got a job at the NWT Brewing Company as a server. They were so short staffed after the pandemic that they hired me even though I had no experience working as a waitress. I thought, if I could stay on my feet and remember people's orders, I could stay on my feet as a nurse too. That was healing for me because it gave me the confidence that my brain and body were fine and that I was going to be okay. The treatment hadn't wreaked havoc on my body. I was really scared I'd come out of treatment and not be able to be a nurse. I'm still working there part-time and can't say enough good things about how the owners accommodated and supported me when I took time off for reconstruction.

I am now in my final semester of nursing school. I have a countdown on my phone for how many days are left until I write my licensing exam. When I think about where I am now when it seemed impossibly hard three years ago, I am filled with a lot of joy and gratitude. So many people helped me and my family navigate through our crisis. Sometimes, something will happen that makes me realize I am still traumatized by everything that happened in 2020 and 2021, but for the most part, I am okay, and my kids are okay too. Since completing cancer treatment, I've ticked some pretty incredible items off my bucket list. In 2023, I drove with my four children from Yellowknife to Calgary, Las Vegas, Disneyland, Laguna Beach, and back again. I got to meet my father in person for the first time in London, United Kingdom. These were all things I dreamed of doing even before I got sick. One really amazing moment was when one of my instructors asked, "Who in this class wants to get their master's degree eventually?" That was my plan before cancer, but hope had become a scary thing, so I barely believed I'd finish the undergraduate program, much less get a master's. However, at that moment, I realized I did believe I would graduate, and I still wanted to be open to graduate studies in the future. So, I put my hand up.

These days, I don't spend much time worrying about the cancer coming back. I've returned to my old strategy of just focusing on the things in my life I have control over. Other than taking my pill every day and getting scans every year, there is not a lot I can do. I devote my energy to things that are important to me, like my kids and school. I'm hoping that in a few years, I can buy a home. After facing housing insecurity during cancer treatment, I never want to experience that again. I am setting mini goals to work towards that larger goal. Every day, my dreams come closer and closer to reality and for that, I am immensely grateful.

Notes

1. In March 2020 the Chief Public Health Officer of the Northwest Territories announced a travel ban. This ban was intended to prevent unnecessary travel and slow the spread of COVID-19. As well, anyone travelling into the Northwest Territories had to isolate for fourteen days upon entry. This included NWT residents who had to leave the territory on medical travel. All NWT COVID-19 Public Health Orders were lifted on April 1, 2022.
2. There is no MRI machine in the Northwest Territories, so patients have to travel South to access this diagnostic test.

Elizabeth (Sabet) Biscaye

YELLOWKNIFE

I am Chipewyan Dene from Rocher River. It's a ghost town now. I grew up on the land until I was about 9 years old, then we moved to Fort Resolution. I did my schooling in Fort Resolution and Fort Smith. My parents had fifteen children all together, seven of us survived and now there's only two of us. Sadly, one of my siblings died from cancer. So, we've had experience with cancer in our family. I have a 42-year-old son who lives in Ontario. He is married with one child. I also have extended family all over the place. I still have a home in Fort Resolution and try to spend as much time there as I can, but I live in Yellowknife for now. When I retire, I hope to move back to Fort Resolution.

I currently work with the territorial government, but I have also worked in other jobs, including with the mining industry, with Indigenous governments across the territories, and with non-profits like the Native Communication Society.[1] We coordinated the development of an action plan for the Missing and Murdered Indigenous Women and Girls report.[2] There is a lot of important work to be done with women and their families. I'm also an interpreter and translator. Languages are my passion. I'm a certified interpreter/translator and have done a lot of interpreting for patients. I often interpreted for my elderly parents when they were still alive. Any time they went to the doctor I would interpret for them. When my father was diagnosed with colon cancer,

I went through his whole journey with him starting from when he got diagnosed to when he had surgery. I learned a lot about colon cancer as I went through that with him. My father made a full recovery but less than a year later he was diagnosed with prostate cancer, which was successfully treated as well. However, that is a story for another time.

After my father's diagnosis, his doctor recommended that all his children get tested because apparently colon cancer can be hereditary. So, we all got colonoscopies done. When I did my colonoscopy, they found some polyps so I was told that I should come back within a couple of years. However, it's not easy to get an appointment. I was on the waiting list for a colon cancer screening test for a long time until I got my family doctor involved and he pestered their offices to get me in for a colonoscopy. I also did a FIT test[3] and they found blood in my stool, so then it became even more urgent.

I was then scheduled for a colonoscopy. I knew what to expect having accompanied my father when he had to have his done. A friend of mine came with me to the appointment. After it was over, I was sitting in the recovery room and the doctor, who was a locum, came in and shoved a picture into my hand and said, "You have a tumour. You're going to need surgery." He could have been a lot more humane when giving me such devastating news. I think that a little bit more of a caring attitude would have certainly made a difference because I was kind of taken aback.

When you're dealing with something like cancer, stress of any sort can really compound. Service providers need to be mindful that cancer patients are already dealing with enough as it is, and medical professionals need to be more sensitive. They need to ask themselves, "If I were in this person's shoes, how would I want to be treated?" Kindness makes a big difference. With the exception of how my diagnosis was shared with me, I was fortunate that all other health personnel that I had dealings with treated me well and with a lot of kindness.

Another thing that helps is knowing every step of the way what is happening with our treatment plans. Having the doctor share instructions with us and being able to provide input into our treatment options make a big difference. The patient might not know things that are going on, and it's not good for doctors to make assumptions. It's better for doctors to be upfront and totally honest about everything with the patient so that way they know what they're dealing with instead of having surprises come up.

All I knew at this point was that there was a tumour in my bowels or in my colon. I had surgery in Yellowknife where they removed half of my colon. There is a medical term for this procedure but don't ask me what it is. I was proud to finally master how to say "colonoscopy" properly, never mind having to remember the medical name for having half my colon removed. I still didn't even know at that point if the tumour was cancerous. It took about a month and a half before I got the diagnosis that it was cancer and that I may need further treatment. My first thought was about my son and my family. I tend to be a very logical person, and I also thought, "What's the next step?"

Keeping in mind that we had recently lost one of my sisters to cancer, I then had to break the news to my family. My family was used to seeing me as a strong, independent person, but now I would need their support. At the time I didn't really think about the implications that breaking the news would have on my family because with my father everything turned out really well, and he survived cancer.

The word "cancer" is scary. Looking back, I feel guilty that I wasn't more sensitive. It was only later on that I thought about it, "Oh my God, I wasn't as sensitive to my family as I should have been." It must have been that much more upsetting for everyone because we had just lost my younger sister to cancer about a year and a half before. I'm the matriarch of the family now after my mother passed away, but even before that I'd always been considered the oldest in the family. So, everybody kind of looks to me for leadership. I think I didn't realize the impact that my cancer had on my family members. I think as cancer patients, we sometimes have to remember the impact on our family and that they may need support too, not just us.

A lot of times people forget about the caregivers because everyone is so focused on the patient. A caregiver's life often revolves around caring so much for the patient that they forget to care for themselves and then depression and other feelings can arise. I remember being in the boarding home in Edmonton when my father was in the hospital, and there was a lady from one of the communities that I shared a room with. She was from the Beaufort Delta[5] and her husband was going through the same surgery as my father. I saw the stress on her face when she would come back at the end of the day just totally wiped. I think it would be very helpful if there was mental health support available for caregivers of cancer patients, even just to chat or have a cup of tea, so that people know they're not alone.

Then again, this whole time I was a caregiver too. Before they did the surgery to remove the tumour there was an infection in my colon that needed to be treated. At that time, I was taking care of my elderly mother and had to make arrangements for her to be cared for. Life doesn't stop for us even when we have cancer. I was very fortunate that my younger sister was able to stay with my mom and take care of her while I was in the hospital.

I was in the hospital for about ten days when a visiting doctor decided to discharge me. It's difficult when locums come in from down South. Physically, I didn't feel like I should be discharged just yet, but I was discharged anyway and instructed to come back in two weeks for a check-up. When I was discharged, arrangements were made for homecare to come and change my dressing as I was still healing. I had been cut open from the bottom of my sternum to past my belly button so there was a large wound to treat. When I went for my follow-up appointment a couple of weeks later, my doctor told me that I had an infection, and I was re-admitted into the hospital for a month and a half. Then I had to have surgery again later on to insert a mesh to make sure I didn't develop a hernia. When I got home, there was an expectation that I was all better. I think my mother thought I could just pick up where I left off, but I was limited in what I could do.

Navigating through day-to-day life and then having to be admitted back into the hospital after having been discharged and then opened up again is a lot to have to go through. The hospital food was not very good, but I needed to eat in order to have strength. When my son was in town, he would sometimes go get me something to eat but of course I also had to be careful of what I ate. It got to the point where I thought of inviting the MLAs[6] to come and share my hospital food with me so they could see for themselves what patients were being asked to eat. I did appreciate the Friday lunches prepared by the Indigenous staff, who also provided interpreting services at the hospital.

It would be really good if there were dedicated mental health support workers available for cancer patients — somebody to talk to when you don't want to talk about what you are going through with your family or your friends because you don't want to worry them. I have a hard time getting people to understand some of the things that have to do with my body. For instance, sometimes I get grumpy with people and I don't mean to. I feel bad but it's because I feel so uncomfortable physically. People don't understand that my internal system has been changed because I look the same on the outside (maybe a few pounds heavier and more wrinkles, ha ha). Even though there were complications to my health, I managed to overcome and adapt to a new way of living.

Our bodies try to adapt to the changes we experience but even when our bodies adapt, we have to be careful. If my bowel movements are not regular, I feel really sluggish and very uncomfortable, and so forth. My belly protrudes now because I've got no working muscles in my abdomen. I was opened three times and they put a mesh in there so there's parts of my body where I have no feeling, or sometimes when I feel itchy around my stomach area, scratching doesn't help. Even though the cancer is gone I'm still dealing with the aftereffects of it and will be for the rest of my life, but I have no problems with that because I think I lucked out. I didn't need chemo and I didn't need to do radiation. They took out the part that had the cancer and I have been cancer free for over five years now, so I am very grateful for that. A couple of people I know went into remission for the same cancer I had. I know of other people who've had the same kind of cancer and lost their lives to it and some who now have to wear a bag for the rest of their life. You never know with cancer.

Having supportive family and friends there with me really made a difference. I was fortunate because I got diagnosed in Yellowknife, where I had family all around me, but I know of people who received the news that they had cancer while they were far away from home. For instance, I was with my late sister in Edmonton when she got her diagnosis that she had lung cancer, and that's something that I would not wish on anybody. The strength and courage I witnessed in my sister in dealing with her cancer was remarkable and admirable. My sister had done some research before she received her diagnosis, so she knew what the prospect for her future was. To carry that kind of burden with dignity and resolve is tremendous. When my sister was going through chemo and radiation treatment, I saw the impact it had on her body and I didn't wish to go through that. When people talk about the "dark side," I think of chemo as the dark side. The chemo and radiation did not stop the cancer from claiming her life, but it did prolong it for a bit.

Since my sister had to be away from home to get treatment, it gave us a chance to build a family of support at the Larga home in Edmonton.[7] We were treated very well at Larga and that made a big difference. Having a lot of Northerners there was also a comfort. We befriended a lot of people there. We did a lot of evening activities together and got to know other people and patients who were dealing with the same thing while far from home. Our family also made sure to call each other on a regular basis. We have to remember that our families back home may be worried about what is happening, so we need to touch base with them and keep them informed. Hearing your loved one's voice provides comfort, too.

When I went out to Edmonton with my sister for her cancer treatment, I had a good job and was getting good pay. We were okay financially, but I noticed other patients down South would sometimes have to take leave from their jobs and if they didn't have benefits, they would lose pay. Even though everything is covered, like meals, you do still need some money to be able to get around. There are ways the community can fundraise to support families, especially if family members are having to travel to support a patient.

One of the things that my parents always instilled in us was that doctors and nurses are there to help you, but you have to help them help you as long as the treatment is reasonable. But still, I found I had to advocate for myself. If I hadn't gotten my family doctor involved, I sometimes wonder, would I have found out I had colon cancer only after it was too late? We hear stories of people in communities where they go undiagnosed for a long time and then when they are finally diagnosed, it's too late. That could have easily been my story because I didn't have any symptoms and I was having trouble getting a follow up. I could have lost my life. Remember: you are the only one who knows how YOU feel. Not even the doctors or nurses know, so you have to speak up for yourself. If you have family members or friends who are helping you, that's good. If you're in one of the smaller communities, the nurses who are familiar with your case should be able to provide ongoing support.

As well, escorts[8] are there to support you. They don't just help get you to appointments. I think with the Indigenous community a lot of times the larger family wants to know what's going on, but patient confidentiality gets complicated so having an escort there to relay information back to anxious family is important. I'm an interpreter so I've been in exam rooms where patients have been told by doctors what the diagnosis is, but patients are sometimes left trying to figure out what kind of cancer they have because they may not understand the medical terminology or what treatment options are available to them, and in those cases it's important to have an escort.

Even with the best efforts of the medical professionals, cancer may change your life in a number of ways, so be prepared for that. You need to respect and listen to your body. My body has been changed physically. My insides are no longer the same as they were before, but that's okay because I'm still alive. I'll make whatever changes I need to keep going. I try to avoid things that are not good for my health. I have to admit, I love my gummy bears, but I am mindful of what I put into my body. I was put on diabetes medication for a while but managed to reverse it, so I didn't need to be on them anymore. Sometimes there's a whole other set of complications that can come up aside from battling cancer.

I did not try traditional Indigenous medicine, not because I don't believe in it but because my father believed that cancer is a new disease to us so it's better to try Western medicine first and if that doesn't work, then try traditional medicine. I thought that was a reasonable approach because I don't think cancer is part of our Indigenous culture, at least not that I know of. I was prepared to go the traditional medicine route if I thought it would help.

The first thing I would do if I found out someone close to me has cancer is I would ask them if they need a hug. It makes a big difference to have human contact, but I know some people are not huggers. I recognize and respect that. Letting them know that they're cared for and that they've got your support is sometimes enough. Some people don't want to say the wrong thing to a cancer patient so they don't say anything. Maybe they are worried they might trigger the person who has cancer. I want to share that it's okay to ask questions, and if they get grumpy with you, just be patient. They're trying to work through some difficult stuff themselves because it's cancer. Even though these days there's a lot of treatment options for cancer, it's still scary. The word cancer used to be so scary. Basically, it was a death sentence. That's not the case anymore. I'm a good example of that. There are a lot of cancers now that can be treated.

But cancer can change a person physically, spiritually, and mentally. It's made me a lot more grateful. I feel blessed that even though I had cancer, I managed to overcome it. I'm still here. It doesn't mean that it's not always in the back of my mind. I think anybody who's ever had cancer will say the same thing. Cancer has taught me a lot of things. It opened my eyes. I got a second chance. I'm not taking anything for granted. I look back on life and the little moments; that's where I find strength. As well, I've always been a spiritual person. I've always believed in the Creator and the power of prayer, and having cancer has made prayer an everyday part of my life. All day, every day, it's in everything I do. I like to believe that the Creator is guiding me and provides me with what I need to deal with any challenges that life throws my way. I've always been like that. I'm grateful to still be here to be able to share my story and I hope it helps provide some comfort to those dealing with cancer. Marsi.

Notes

1. Native Communications Society has been in operation since 1982. The organization runs CKLB radio, which broadcasts throughout the Northwest Territories and to some communities in Alberta. On their website, they share "we provide the most amount of Dene language programming in the world".
2. The National Inquiry on Missing and Murdered Indigenous Women and Girls released their final report and 231 Calls for Justice in 2019. Entitled, "Reclaiming Power and Place," it can be read at https://www.mmiwg-ffada.ca/. The action plan developed by the GNWT was tabled in 2021.
3. FIT stands for fecal immunochemical test. It is used to detect small amounts of blood in someone's stool.
4. The Beaufort Delta, "Beau Del," or just "the Delta" is the region in northwestern Northwest Territories where the Mackenzie Delta eventually reaches the Arctic Ocean. It's the ancestral home to Inuvialuit and Gwich'in Peoples.
5. Members of the Legislative Assembly. Northwest Territories and Nunavut are the only territorial or provincial jurisdictions in Canada with a consensus government. That means there are no political parties at the territorial level, and government makes decisions by consensus.
6. Larga Homes are boarding homes for Northern medical travellers. There are Larga Homes in the Edmonton area (Leduc), Yellowknife, and Ottawa.
7. A medical travel escort is someone who is able to accompany a patient on medical travel. This is a role that is approved and has expenses covered by the NTHSSA through medical travel.

Stephen Buchanan

YELLOWKNIFE

I'm about to turn 63. I had rectal cancer. My sphincter was removed. I have a colostomy bag. I am currently waiting for hip surgery.

I've lived all over Canada. I've been in Yellowknife for twenty years. My reaction when I found out I had cancer was not very good. I went to the oncologist. There were four sections on the report she dealt with. The first three were fine but on the fourth one she said I had cancer. I felt it was unfair that she didn't tell me right away. I'd rather know. I was supposed to work that night and I phoned my boss and said, "I can't work." I was a bartender at the time. I was devastated. The doctor was relatively empathetic. She has a hard job telling people they have cancer. I wasn't shocked. I kind of figured it was coming.

I don't really like the term survivor. I didn't want to play the cancer card saying to those closest to me, "I'm dying from cancer." I tried to minimize it. My family is back in Toronto but I'm really close with my sister, and when I told her she started crying. Mostly, I told my close friends here in Yellowknife. They were realistic about what I was going through and that was helpful. My friends got together and supported me. They were unbelievably supportive and that was incredible. Crystal Fraser, Jenna Snow, and Sandy Craig started a community fundraiser and raised

Photo by Terry Hartwright.

$16,000. I didn't do taxes for twenty years and I got back $20,000 when I finally did my taxes, and that helped with being off work.

I ended up doing most of my chemotherapy treatment at the Cross Cancer Institute in Edmonton. My friend Crystal Fraser, who is a prof at the University of Alberta, was there with me every day, so I had really good support. It was really disturbing getting treatment. I would see little 8-year-old kids with no hair and that disturbed me. Having an escort with me in Edmonton was quite helpful, but the last time I flew down I didn't get a travel buddy. When I had an escort, it was hugely helpful because I'm not the most organized guy.

I smoke and I drink. I don't really look after my body. I think I got cancer because of my unhealthy lifestyle. I eat more now. I eat better. I was so scrawny when I got out of the hospital. I'm down to a pack and half of cigarettes a day. I still drink. I'm in a lot of pain because of my hip. For the last ten years I've been trying to get hip surgery. I'm worried about getting addicted to opioids, so I don't take drugs for the pain. I used to be a competitive cyclist — riding long distances and training intensely — which often resulted in broken or bruised ribs. I've learned how to live with pain. The easy way out is taking opioids, and I don't want to do the easy way out. With that being said, if they told me there was no chance to live otherwise, then I would take the drugs. But right now I refuse to take drugs.

I'm a bit of a depressive, naturally. I feel almost negatively about having cancer. I have a colostomy bag that's attached to me for the rest of my life. I've lost my sphincter. I don't like that there's an alien object attached to me, but the alternative is that I'm dead. I don't know how long I'll be alive. I don't think much longer. You've got to be realistic about this. I think a lot more about mortality now that I've had cancer. My dad died of a brain tumour when he was 54. Aside from him and myself, there is no cancer in our family.

I was just at the doctor and she said my heart was strong. When getting the call that says, "You've got cancer," some people can roll over and die and some can choose to live. I might live for another twenty years. I don't know if there's a right way to say it, but just make sure you have family and friends and you'll do all right.

~

In memory of Stephen Buchanan, May 14, 1960 to September 23, 2023

Allice Legat

YELLOWKNIFE

In 2018 I went to the doctor for pink eye that wouldn't go away. The doctor — a locum — heard rattling in my lungs. I insisted it was my asthma. After all, asthma could have been the reason. I was so tired, which is a symptom of the dust allergy that triggered my asthma. But the doctor thought I may have pneumonia, so off I went for an x-ray. He called me with the results, starting with, "You may have…" And I interrupted saying, "Cancer." I'm still not exactly sure why I said that, but probably because my mum died of lung cancer, my grandma of leukaemia, and an uncle of brain cancer; it just made sense when he started with *you may have*. He responded, "Yes, but we won't know for sure until you have more tests." I quickly asked, "I have a chance to go to Barrow, Alaska, next week. Can I still go?" He said, "The tests will not be scheduled for at least a week, and if it's cancer, what difference will it make if you travel? And if it's pneumonia, I've given you medication." So off I went, days after telling Jacob, my son, and Maggy, my daughter-in-law, about the probability of cancer. My desire to take the Barrow trip to listen to Elders talk about their desire for their own university, as well as eat whale after seeing where it was stored deep in the permafrost, was more powerful than my fear of experiencing the same pain my mother had as she slipped away from us.

Photo by Tessa MacIntosh Photography.

I've lived in Yellowknife since 1986. I was born in Saskatchewan and raised in Alberta. When I came to the place of the Dene — after working and travelling in many places in the world — I felt at home. I love being in Denendeh, as the Dene call their homeland, which encompasses most of the Northwest Territories. I really enjoy the openness of the people that I meet here. I have worked mainly with the Tłı̨chǫ Dene since the early 1990s. Their stories tell me their history, values, and struggles through time, and about whose land I live on. My Scottish grandfather always emphasized the importance of knowing whose traditional land you live on. So here I am, in 2025, living here, with stage 4 lung cancer.

My first trip to Edmonton to determine if I had cancer or not was in March 2018. Tests were done at both the Royal Alexandra Hospital and the Cross Cancer Institute. My son made the trip with me. The tests included an ECG for my heart, and MRI, CT, and PET scans to determine if and where the cancer may be. We flew home, and just as I was unpacking my suitcase, they called me and wanted me back the next day: my cancer had metastasized, which surprised everyone, and a biopsy was critical to getting me on treatment as soon as possible. My son travelled with me back to the Royal Alexandra, where they had a bed for me. I couldn't have my upper right lobe removed; I couldn't have radiation. I had to have a biopsy to determine the marker of my cancer, so they'd know how to treat me.

I was surprised that the surgeon could weave through my ribs to access a location where a mass to analyze could be taken from my pleura. At first, I thought I could only have chemo, but as Lung Cancer Canada[1] explained when I called them, I could ask about a clinical trial. And the Lung Cancer Canada staff emphasized that I make sure the surgeon took enough pathological material during the biopsy so my oncologist, Dr. Butts, could determine if it matched the markers of any of the clinical trials. I wasn't even presented with these trials until the biopsy cuts were healed. That took six weeks, and then I waited for a clinical trial that was studying a treatment in relation to my exact type of cancer. My treatment started four months after suspecting cancer and three months after my biopsy. The clinical test that I agreed to was a randomized trial to evaluate the safety and effect of the combination of immunotherapy, in lung cancer patients, with or without standard chemotherapy.

I started treatment in May 2018 with durvalumab and tremelimumab (the immunotherapy drugs) along with standard doses of chemotherapy every three weeks. After seven months, treatment was every four weeks. After three years, when the side effects became too numerous and my cancer was stable, I was taken off the study and observed every three months, and now every four months. My cancer has been still for over two years. As of March 14, 2023, I have lived with stage 4 lung cancer for five years. I am one of the lucky ones; only 5 percent of stage 4 lung cancer patients survive five years compared to the 22 percent who are diagnosed earlier and compared to 91 percent of those with prostate cancer, 89 percent with breast cancer, and 67 percent with colorectal cancer.

These discrepancies are due to a lack of research into lung cancer. I personally don't see any cancer as worse than any other. Anyone can get cancer, including lung cancer; any animal can get cancer. The problem is we haven't done enough research on certain kinds of cancer.

Cancer affects everyone around you, all your friends and family. Jacob, Maggy, and I had bought a plot of land before I was diagnosed. My son designed a home for them with a suite for me, but he had to give up that dream so they could care for me. Jacob researched the drugs I was on, healthy food I should eat, and protein drinks I could get down; he knew that I didn't want to eat or drink anything containing preservatives. And Maggy searched for a home we could all enjoy. They both read all the information I had to make decisions on. The lot was eventually sold. A home was found, and Jacob, friends, and contractors renovated the suite to be more suitable for me.

Initially, I wanted to tell only my family and friends I had lung cancer because it's viewed by the public as being one's own fault. I didn't want people asking me if I smoked, and I didn't want to explain again and again that there are many reasons why people and animals get lung cancer and smoking is only one reason. I learned the stats when my mother was ill, so I've always known one in three people will get some kind of cancer in their lifetime. But now it is one in two, with 82 Canadians being diagnosed with lung cancer every day.

I have found that being actively involved in any health issue impacting me has always been a helpful way to deal with any associated fear and anxiety. And I now know that lung cancer is the most diagnosed and leading killer of all cancers in Canada; approximately 21,000 people died with it in 2022. Now I'm starting to join groups that advocate for regular CT scans for all people so people will be diagnosed before it has metastasized to other parts of their bodies, allowing people to be cured more effectively. And I try, especially during November, lung cancer month, to set up a table at the Yellowknife Direct Charge Co-op so I can share information with others. Whether I do it or not depends on my health.

At first, as I said above, I did not want my loved ones to tell people I had cancer; however, I soon realized that that was selfish. All people who care for cancer patients also need care; they need to talk about what their loved ones are going through. I learned this as I saw my cancer hurt others emotionally. I saw how they responded. Each person responds differently to their own cancer and to the cancer of a family member or friend. When I told my son and daughter-in-law at the Woodyard, Yellowknife's local brew pub, over a half pint of beer on a Friday night, I heard silence, and then we discussed the signs that now made sense, especially my tiredness. Everyone I know who had or has cancer is tired. For me, that also meant eating too much trying to get more energy, therefore gaining unhealthy fat, as well as falling due to being tired and out of shape. People think the signs of cancer are pain, yet, to me, a common sign for all I have known before they were diagnosed with cancer is tiredness. It is not us being "just lazy" or "just getting old."

Maggy, Jacob, and I sat discussing cancer in a logical way at the pub. We were not our usual teasing and debating selves, and I could see fear and concern in my son's face and Maggy's concern for Jacob and me. I called my sister Rossanne and heard silent weeping. She had been the main caregiver for Mum, as they had both lived in Calgary. And, since my friend Joanne was in town, I told her over coffee at my home. She burst into tears as so many people she has known have died of cancer, and she said, "We have more to do together." I can't remember when I told Pat, a friend who had had cancer, but she told me that after ten years she still worries cancer will take over her life again. And Debbie, who is very logical with a no-nonsense approach, immediately helped me to navigate the medical system. I will never forget that so many people brought me laughter, hugs, as well as food, like berries, fish, boreal caribou, and moose. I was spoiled. People from Gamètì gave me beaded caribou pouches containing medicine from the land.

My sister and her 90-year-old husband came to Edmonton to be with me during my very difficult time in 2018. And during the same year, my niece Stacie came from Calgary, to support me, and she, along with her 10-year-old son Seran, travelled to Yellowknife to spend time with me and give Jacob and Maggy a break. I was so fatigued and emotionally distant from myself that I was short and rude without realizing it. They all stood by me.

With every type of cancer, families suffer, the caregivers suffer, and the patient watches those they love go through agony. They are strong for us, and they are being challenged emotionally for our sake. Not only did I need a counsellor who understood cancer fear, but caregivers also need counsellors. None of my family could find good ones in the Northwest Territories. I am still looking.

After a few treatments I started having side effects. They slowly got worse. I was in and out of emergency, falling and passing out. Once I passed out and fell off the toilet, only waking sometime later to find I was bruised down one side and had a headache due to my head landing on the floor tiles. This time of my life was horrifying for me, and I'd like to share a story I wrote about it.

The Monster That Crawls

Up the elevator to the treatment room, called the Penthouse because the large windows allow patients and their caregivers to watch the birds land on the tree-covered landscape and feel the sun warming them, giving them hope. The sequence of drugs trickle into my veins for five and a half hours every three weeks for the clinical trial at the Cross Cancer Institute. I don't fall asleep like the other patients. My caregiver — always a different family member or friend — laughs with me, challenges me with questions like, do I think most cancer is a by-product of aging? Will we ever have clean energy? Or more often we discuss restaurants, trying to find one especially relaxing to visit after my treatment. I don't lose my life as others do. But I slowly lose my mind as I give in to the drip, drip, drip, and smiling faces of the research staff.

I notice my mind going when I can no longer share my thoughts. They call it chemo fog. I know it is not just living in a fog; there's a sensation like an insect crawling along and blocking my synapses, then my words stop, but my mind continues. I never know when it will happen or for how long.

I breathe in the richness of the air inside The Silk Road Spice Merchant on Whyte Avenue. I approach a salesclerk with brown hair, a nose ring, and pale lips. I want to ask for pink peppercorns, but all I can do is open my mouth and make grunting sounds. The young woman, whose face tightens in a mixture of shock, fear, and repulsion, quickly composes herself. I'm sorry for scaring her but can say nothing, so I leave the shop downcast, slowly walking back over the eight blocks to Compassion House for women with cancer who live outside of Edmonton. I know that no one there, not staff or guests, will see me as dysfunctional and unstable; all the cancerous women at the house are trying to make sense of what's happening to their bodies and minds. They don't pity each other; they listen, cry, and laugh together, but they don't pity. Nevertheless, I want to hide from them. I go to the second floor and sit by the gas fireplace, watching magpies as they bother squirrels, and only when my voice returns do I go down and make dinner.

I try to blank out the terror of losing my cognitive abilities. I hope to push myself to go through the motions of living a normal life.

But normalcy isn't possible. I can't find my words, or even utter a sound, to answer a question after my presentation at an environmental monitoring conference back home in the Northwest Territories. The facilitator calls a break to give me time to compose myself. Almost everyone thinks it's nerves, and they are somewhat correct, yet only a few know it's the monster that travels my body, disabling the impulses between nerves in my brain. Another time, my friend Dave visits and when I open my mouth I can't speak my thoughts. Nothing comes out, not even the grunts and groans of the spice shop. I see his fear-filled eyes as he sits semi-paralyzed, wondering what to do, wanting to help. Then he stands as if wanting to hug me but instead gently touches my arm, walks calmly up the stairs, and escapes through the door.

I guess many cancer patients see the same pity, fear, and confusion in others. People witness our silence and numbness as we blank out thoughts of a fast death, or perhaps a painfully slow death, at the same time as we experience the not-so-pleasant side effects of treatments that just might save our lives. My family and close friends do not reduce me to a woeful person: they tease me, help me laugh, bring life back to my spirit.

The last time I felt the crawling is a sunny spring day. I try to call my friend Debbie before the monster takes over. I want to go to emergency while it's happening, I want medical professionals to tell me what's happening.

I feel my mind shut down. I know the thing that crawls has won. I can see Debbie's phone number in my mind's eye but can't connect the numbers with the digits on my cell. If I can find the "four," the other numbers will follow. They don't, because I can't figure out which number is four! It could be any of them. I try to print "4," but I can't. I decide to get dressed while my mind is blocked. I know what I want to wear, I know what my jeans look like; that is all in my mind, but as I peer at them, all my clothes look like jeans. I can't even dress. I sob uncontrollably for a moment, then sit on the floor, leaning against the wall and clutching the low windowsill for an hour, maybe more, watching birds whose names I know but can't speak. Finally, I feel my mind release and a flood of electrical flashes reach my mouth; I spit out their names: eagle, robin, warbler, raven.

I quickly punch in Debbie's number on my cell. She answers, but before I can tell her I need to go to emergency, my synapses are once again disabled. Debbie doesn't know what's happening; she asks me if I need a latte from Birchwood, and just like in the spice shop I grunt like a mad beast. Calmly as Debbie can, she says she's coming over. She arrives and all I can do is point at my bare legs and babble. Debbie laughs that I have only sweaters and t-shirts on my bed, she finds my jeans and I slip into them, she hands me a brown long-sleeve t-shirt I pull over my head.

In the car I gaze out the window at the puny, stunted spruce trees growing from tiny bits of earth on the bedrock; I enjoy spotting a small stream flowing over the steep cliff where it brightens the red of the iron deposits showing through the substratum. Without realizing I'm speaking, I say, "The red is so vibrant today." Shocked, I exclaim, "I'm back!"

After checking in at emergency, we are told to wait outside until one of the private rooms is free, so that I will be away from the potentially contagious people in the waiting room. As we sit outside, away from the wheelchair smokers, a police officer leads away a patient whose hands are cuffed and ankles are chained together.

I'm taken to a private room where the bed is attached to the floor in the centre of the room; I must squat down to the foot-high bed. There are no chairs and no other furniture. A camera is high in a corner. It's all very strange. The room is usually reserved for criminals with violent behaviour, but today it is for me and my sketchy immune system. I giggle to myself, hoping they do not chain me to the heavy link in the floor if the monster awakens and slithers.

I have a CT scan and am told there is nothing wrong with my brain. The doctor on call patiently spends an hour chatting with me, learning that I also fall for no reason and there is an ugly rash on my right leg. My oncologist, Dr. Butts, is contacted. Chemo may be the culprit.

During my next visit to the Cross in Edmonton, Dr. Butts recommends that two drugs be stopped, reducing the drip, drip to an hour's worth of one drug, durvalumab, every four weeks. I struggle with giving up the combination of chemo and immunotherapy because it did shrink the tumour and nodules, and I want them to shrink even more, but I also want to be rid of the thing that crawls.

I chose to accept the changes to my treatment, and I'm back to myself. Now the clinical trial is over. I am stable, living with cancer that sits quietly. When people ask me what the disconnect felt like, I usually say little; I don't want to think about what dementia may be like. The monster that slithered may be gone, and I do dread it may crawl and terrorize me again. I also know I will do it all again, when necessary.

My friend Joanne and I sat for hours in the multi-faith room at the Cross, where I was trying to decide whether to go off or stay on chemo. We sat there touching the beautiful stones in a bowl. I've always liked the feel of small, smooth stones. Let me remind you I wanted the tumours and nodules to continue shrinking. I feared going off chemo.

Joanne said, "Let's pray, Allice." I told her, "I know how to pray, but mostly I just like to think about who I want to talk to, and I'd rather talk to my ancestors." So, I started thinking about all the older people who had told me stories and all those who, when alive, provided me with guidance and support. After a few minutes she asked, "Who are you talking to?" and I said, "Everyone is rushing in." We looked at each other and burst out laughing as she said, "Well, you might never get an answer." Grandpa Campbell, who played the fiddle while Mum did the Scottish fling and tapped, and Romie Wetrade, a maker of drums, both showed themselves. They were directing me to dance.

We went back to our hotel room, and Joanne used her phone to find music for us to dance to on YouTube. We danced to the fiddle music I grew up with and to the Dene drums that have become part of my current life. We laughed as I could barely lift my feet as I danced. I talked to my sister and Jacob about the decision. They both told me they would support whatever I decided. Joanne found music; first we two-stepped, then we danced to the drums. We laughed more than we danced; I could barely move as I held on to Joanne. Then answers came. I needed to get off the chemo. I received the guidance I wanted. I have great people around me both in this world and in the spirit world.

I believe it was during this period that Joanne found Sorrentino's Compassion House.[2] Staying at the hotel was eating up all my savings, and during that trip I had to wait for treatment but I was too sick and I couldn't get off the couch — I just lay there shivering even though it was 29° Celsius in my room. I stayed in Edmonton for twenty days waiting to be well enough for treatment.

At Compassion House and as soon as I could sit up for more than a minute, Joanne insisted I walk up and down stairs. No elevator for me. I'd told all my caregivers I wanted to stay strong. Joanne, being Dene, would always make a massive amount of food for me and others in the house. She still insists that good food, as well as physical activities, keeps us strong. Pat and I walked Whyte Avenue together, exploring shops, movies, and the theatres. More than once she, like the others, had to carry everything and balance me after a treatment. Family and friends all escorted me to Edmonton for treatment until COVID-19 hit and I started traveling every four weeks alone. Jacob, when not in a meeting, listened on his cell phone to my discussions with my oncologist, especially when decisions had to be made, and when he couldn't, Pat listened and took notes.

During COVID the support was gone while the fear associated with my CT scans increased. Two things helped: My nephew Miles picked me up and delivered me back to the airport so I would not have to be in taxis or shuttles; and staying at Compassion House, where women visited, talked, and laughed, all while wearing masks.

When I'm scared, I'm all over the place like a nitwit. Since cancer, I deal with fear by walking, cooking, reading about what's happening to me, and writing stories, all of which calm me down. People praise me for doing so well but, on the inside, just before my CT scans, I'm scared, despite being stable for the last two years. Other cancer patients now in remission tell me they still fear the cancer returning. Sometimes I feel fortunate as I already know I will be living with cancer forever, but my fear is that it will start growing again.

As you may or may not know, during the COVID-19 pandemic, cancer patients being treated in Edmonton and living in the Northwest Territories had to isolate for two weeks after returning home. By the time the public health orders were lifted, I was isolated for thirty weeks in total. Jacob brought food and left it at my door, Maggy gave me a gratitude book to write down three good things that happened every day, and my friend Dana put together a book called *Covid Cocktails* and hung it on my doorknob, causing me to laugh out loud. Others also left food and trinkets at my door.

Nevertheless, after thirty weeks I found that I didn't want to get dressed, I didn't want to go outside, I kept saying I'll do it tomorrow. So, I wrote about it and called the story "Da Capo al Fine" which is "to repeat" in music, or one week in Edmonton, two weeks in isolation, one week keeping a two-metre distance from everyone. I found isolation hard and couldn't imagine what it was like for cancer patients from other communities in the Northwest Territories who had to isolate in a Yellowknife hotel before returning to their home — or choosing not to go for treatment because they have no childcare. At times I felt guilty; I knew it was probably easier for me.

I've experienced so many conflicted feelings through my cancer journey. I experienced joy when friends became cancer free; gratitude towards my friends and family. I experienced anguish like never before when a young woman, on the same clinical trial as me, had tumours that were rapidly growing even as mine were shrinking. We visited as she lay dying in the University Hospital while she wondered how she'd say good-bye to her young son. I just listened, then went home and wept.

Through all this I have learned that we really are just human and we do not know how we will behave when we hear we have cancer, or when we hear a loved one has cancer, or when we hear anyone has cancer.

When appropriate I hug someone when I find out they have cancer, but it depends on the situation. Often it is the caregiver who wants and needs a hug, so I hug them, and gently touch the cancerous person who needs to just hold themselves together. I try to listen, but like many of my caregivers, I can, at times, get bossy, telling them what to eat and not eat. I try not to. I often buy people cookbooks designed for cancer patients, so they have hints on what to put in their bodies, like fish.

My heart cries when people tell me they have cancer, when people die of cancer — not so much for them but for myself and the ones who must live without them.

I never tell people with cancer they're going to be okay because we don't know, and I would never want anyone to say that to me. Rather, I encourage people to call me any time they want to talk, morning or night.

I'm pretty sure I will die of lung cancer but in the meantime, I am looking forward to finishing the book I am currently writing, and I would dearly love to visit all my friends, everywhere.

Notes

1. Lung Cancer Canada is a resource for education, patient support, research, and advocacy.
2. Compassion House provides safe, comfortable, and affordable accommodations in Edmonton for women who must leave their homes for cancer care.

Patrick Scott

YELLOWKNIFE

I came North in 1975 as a contract cameraman for CBC to cover the Berger Inquiry for the Mackenzie Valley pipeline.[1] I worked with a great team of Indigenous reporters. It was quite profound. During that time, I met Gabrielle Mackenzie from Behchokǫ̀. We married and had eight children, six girls and two boys. We now have fourteen grandchildren. I've really built a strong sense of family, community, and great relationships with so many people. I feel so honoured by what the North has given to me, and I hope in some ways I can give back because I've been so well treated.

In 2012 I had a bad cold that wouldn't go away. My youngest daughter, Jawah, made a doctor's appointment for me. I didn't want to go but because she made that appointment I went. As a result of that doctor's visit, I was diagnosed with prostate cancer.

I had a lot of symptoms, including fatigue and a painful sensation when urinating, but like a lot of men I ignored them. I brushed it off as, "Well, I'm getting older and I guess this comes with age." Cancer didn't enter my thoughts at all. In some respects, it came as a surprise but when I started educating myself on the symptoms, I thought that it was pretty stupid of me not to recognize something was wrong with my health.

After that first doctor's visit I informed my family that I probably had cancer. Then I went out to Edmonton for a biopsy and a week later it was confirmed. My kids are kind of spread all around. We are not all in the same community, so I had a conference call with them. I called them all at the same time and we went from there. In the spring of 2013, I went to Edmonton for radiation treatment. I had two months of daily treatment for prostate cancer. That's when my cancer journey began.

We all have our own gut reaction, and I can tell you that for me there was certainly fear when I found out I had cancer. You start saying to yourself, "Is this going to be my last birthday? Is this going to be my last Christmas?" Those emotions well up and you start working on getting past the fear to deal with the reality of treatment and aftercare. Quite honestly, I found that the most important part of aftercare was the love and support of family and friends, which is so energizing. It really makes a huge difference because you don't know where this journey is going to take you and how long the journey is going to continue.

Things were good for me until 2016, and then my cancer metastasized. Since then, I've had ongoing treatment and personal evaluation of how to live with cancer. The ongoing treatment for metastasized prostate cancer is not difficult to take, but it is difficult to live with. I had to get an injection every three months and the side effects were horrendous. That aspect of cancer has been the most difficult; the treatment really impacts quality of life. I am on a continuous roller coaster of high days and down days. Some days it seems bleak and dark. In those times family has been so important. I don't know how people who don't have good relationships have the courage to continue the journey. If you have people around you that you care about, that's a great motivation to keep going and stay as healthy as possible. It's been ten years now since I had my initial cancer treatment.

The cancer continued to spread even with the hormone treatments. In 2023 I was told I had stage 4a cancer, which means the prostate cancer had spread to my pelvic lymph nodes. I was prescribed another subversion drug to take daily. But these drugs don't kill the cancer. After doing some research I found a treatment that wasn't available in Canada. I had to go to Germany to receive a treatment called Lu177 PSMA therapy. It kills the cancer cells. The treatment is ongoing as I write this, but there is a reduction of cancer and it hasn't spread further.

The love and care of others and the fulfilment that it can bring to you is really, really vital. That's what keeps me going. It gives me reason to want to have a good day. I visit my grandchildren and it fills my heart with joy and I say, "Well, cancer isn't going to beat me. Even if it kills me, it's not going to beat me because my spirit is going to remain strong."

Throughout one's lifetime there are often traumatic events that we face that often make us angry. We all have our triggers and if something triggers us, it can come out as anger. Cancer sort of escalates everything because you are wondering how much longer you have. Some people get angry and say, "Why me?" I've never gone down that road. If you start feeling angry, you've got to find a way to let that go. Anger doesn't build goodness. It doesn't bring hope. It's a destructive feeling. You have to find ways to heal yourself from your anger and get rid of your resentment. Don't ask, "Why me?" Ask instead, "What can I do to make my day better?" or "What can I do to make the lives of those around me better?" It's about taking the best from inside yourself, reaching out, and trying to care for others. That's what gives you strength and courage to keep going.

I'm still in hormone suppression therapy and it really has devastated me physically, emotionally, and, in some ways, spiritually. The physical reality is that it causes sleep deprivation, bone pain, sweating spells, and skin rashes. The particular medication I'm on can increase the risk of heart failure. The accumulation of side effects leads to other health issues. One of the things I developed is a cognitive disorder which can lead to dementia or Alzheimer's if it's not dealt with. With the help of my doctor, I've sought alternate treatment outside of the normal medical system with naturopaths and immunologists. We monitor my prostate specific antigen (PSA) levels regularly. As long as my PSA levels stay down, I don't take the injection. I take supplements to help keep the PSA levels down. A daily diet of tomatoes is good because studies show they have a number of chemicals that help suppress PSA. This tomato journey I'm on is a new experiment for me, and it's a new way of instilling hope.[2] I'm trying all kinds of things. I take a lot of vitamins and mineral supplements because cancer also attacks your calcium. It's a nuisance to take all of these pills every day — I've been doing it for six years now — but it helps. So much of our health is about our body being in a balanced state. My immunologist says it's all chemistry.

I think our diets have a huge impact on making us vulnerable to cancer. In the research that I've done our diets play such a big role in the development of cancers within us. Some of it might be environmental but probably more than anything it's genetics and diet. There's an old expression, "we are what we eat," and if we don't look after what we eat then our bodies have to fight what we put in and that enables things like cancer and other diseases to come in and weaken our immune systems.

When I first had cancer, I used different traditional medicines. I've gone to sweats and traditional healers. Part of the challenge is figuring out the best dose. Healing is unique to you. A certain type of traditional medicine can be really helpful and make a difference for one person and for another it might not work. I've tried chaga from the birch tree and I drink dandelion tea. I reduce my carbs and sugars, which is really important because cancer loves those things. In my view you should try everything you can over and beyond what the medical system provides because you don't know what's going to work. I'm quite willing to try anything and everything. I tried CBD oil for about six months, too. Personally, I didn't see any results, but I have friends that have used it and have had good results. You don't give up. You keep trying to find the right solution. I'm sure there are solutions that we still need to discover.

One of the worst parts of my journey was that the doctor was abrupt and unemphatic when telling me I had cancer, then forgot to refer me to the Cross Cancer Institute for treatment. After months of waiting one of my daughters got on the phone and discovered that he forgot to refer me. When I did eventually go to the Cross Cancer Institute, my experience was good. Most of the workers there are good, caring, and sensitive caregivers, but I did have a couple of nurses that were kind of cranky. My current family doctor has been incredible; she's really supportive and willing to explore all kinds of possibilities, including advising me on self-care. The specialists I have seen have not been the best. A couple of them were good, but if it wasn't for my family doctor it would have been a difficult journey. What has been made very clear is that you have to advocate for yourself in the medical system. You can't rely on somebody else giving you the information you need. If you can't do it yourself, you have to have somebody advocating for you. Someone to ask the questions, get the information, and do the research. It's so important. I would urge anyone who is facing cancer to be very proactive in learning about it, question the diagnosis, question the proposed treatment plan, look at all the possibilities for treatment, and do not rule anything out.

Seek out as much advice from every level of expert. You can't rely on just one doctor to tell you everything.

Also, medical travel does a poor job of looking after patients. For example, meal allowances given to a person on medical travel compared to the meal allowance a government worker gets when on duty travel is embarrassing. It's inappropriate. When I went on medical travel, I got $18 a day for meals and $50 per day for private accommodation. A government worker in 2023 got $128.95 per day for meals alone.[3] It's not right. There's something wrong in the system when there's such a disparity. It's something that needs to be addressed.

When you start struggling with the emotions that cancer brings, you have to work on finding peace. Finding peace means letting go, and letting go means forgiving yourself. If you can't be at peace with yourself then peace won't be a part of who you are. Forgiving yourself is part of it. Forgiving others is too. We live in a time where we talk about reconciliation. You have to be willing to forgive if you want to be healthy, and that's not always easy to do. We need to grateful for the good things that are in our lives and for the struggles because that's where we learn and grow. We learn more from the struggle than the comfort — that's human nature.

Cancer is one of those things that teaches us. I have a friend who was diagnosed with cancer and probably won't live much longer, and here I am living with cancer for more than ten years. I think cancer still has a lot to teach me, so I better keep learning from it. I don't feel guilty about my time being longer than my friend's time. I see it as my friend has learned the lessons of life more quickly than I have. I'm surviving because I still have lots to learn before I pass into the spirit world. Cancer is a preparation time for that passing. Gratitude is what keeps me going. I humbly say that I've always had a strong faith, but cancer helped deepen that faith. The Creator is present in our lives both personally and collectively as a community. The Creator is in all creation and our challenge is to constantly recognize the Creator's presence and honour it in ourselves, others, and the world around us. Facing cancer certainly helps you focus on the presence of Creator. For me, my faith and my spiritual journey is as important as anything and it is very sustaining. It helps me get rid of those negative parts of myself in attitude and expressions. It helps me forgive myself and others and be grateful.

You have to make yourself let go of pressures and stress and loneliness. It doesn't matter where you are, whether you're in your own home surrounded by your family or in a hotel room in another city when you're getting treatment, you can experience overwhelming loneliness. That can be very real and powerful, and it can drag you down. You have to simply take time to breathe and say to yourself, "My life isn't just about cancer" or "My life isn't just about being financially stressed." Then look towards the positive things in your life whether it's a grandchild, a meal that you're sitting down to eat, or an ice cream cone. It's as simple as that. Start focusing on being grateful for the good things in your life. It will allow you to walk away from that darkness one step at a time through refocusing your attention.

Since having cancer, I wonder if a knee ache is cancer or if it's just arthritis. Is it going to take me down? That worry is constant because you don't know what the next expression of cancer is going to be when you've had metastasized cancer. Don't focus on that or it will drag you down into the pit. You have to refocus on redirecting your thinking to the positive instead of the negative. It has so much to do with how you see yourself and how you relate to others. It's not about pretending it isn't there. That's not the solution. The solution is accepting it, but not letting it control you.

Being present when engaging with those who are facing cancer and not being afraid to talk about it is important. I know people who get cancer and sort of go into a hole and stay there. Encourage people who have cancer to talk about it, to tell their story, because storytelling is healing. It helps us heal. It not only helps us heal; it helps inform others. Something positive that's happened in my journey might help someone else. Community members can be great listeners if they remain present and curious enough to have the courage to say to somebody, "So, what's going on? I hear you have cancer. Tell me about it." It's a simple question. It doesn't have to be a complex or imposing question. It's just a simple question, but it's really valuable to be able to ask that question and listen carefully to what answer you get.

Some things are hard and some things are easy. Cancer is part of the hard journey so face it head on. You're not alone. At the beginning it feels very lonely and scary, so you need to do your research. Learn as much as you can about what you're going through. Don't just live with it. Learn about it. Don't depend on doctors to be your teachers; learn on your own and have someone help you if you need to. The access we have to information is incredible, so make use of it. Recognize that you are going to be afraid and angry, and then figure out how to deal with it. Don't let those feelings fester and control you.

Notes

1. The Berger Inquiry, also called the Mackenzie Valley Pipeline Inquiry, was led by Justice Thomas Berger beginning in March 1971 to investigate the social, environmental, and economic impacts of a proposed gas pipeline that would run through the Mackenzie River valley in the Northwest Territories. This was a watershed event in the Northwest Territories: the commission visited all communities that would be affected to gauge public reaction. The Inquiry gave full voice to Indigenous Peoples about the lands the pipelines would traverse, and how their cultures and ways of life would be affected.
2. After his interview, Patrick's PSA levels jumped up significantly. His tomato experiment didn't work well enough to prevent having another injection, but he says he will keep trying different experiments.
3. Government of the Northwest Territories employees and eligible dependents receive additional benefits above and beyond the support provided to all NWT residents. In addition to increased funds for accommodations and meals, GNWT employees also have support from benefits officers in human resources who are able to help book travel, hotel, car rental, and process expenses.

Rueben Unka

YELLOWKNIFE

I am originally from Fort Resolution. I just turned 51 when I was diagnosed with cancer and it's been four years. Cancer kind of snuck up on me. I had quit smoking but started spitting blood. I asked about it and some people said, "Well, you quit smoking and it could be because of that," so I just let it go for about a month. But then it got a little bit worse, so I went to the doctor and they sent me out for tests. He called me after and told me that I had cancer. It hit me and terrified me for a few seconds. But then right away he said, "But…" When he said that it was like cold water, and I could breathe. He said, "In the next couple of weeks you'll be on a plane to Edmonton, and it will be removed." As soon as he told me I had cancer, I thought about chemo and losing my hair and weight. I don't have much weight to begin with. Within two weeks I was on a plane down to Edmonton. It was removed, and I was cancer free.

Losing part of my lung made it hard to move around, like walking up the hill to the Explorer Hotel where I had to stay in isolation for COVID. I had to stop three times. Now I'm fine. The doctor said within a year I would be back to normal. I did smoke all my life so I couldn't run around the block to begin with anyway. Now I'm back to where I was, but I do lose my breath sometimes. If I'm walking and talking, I can't do both. If I get a bit of excitement and anxiety, it does affect my breathing.

The operation itself was a laparoscopy, so I wasn't cut open. They put tubes through my throat and my back and took it out slowly that way, but it did do some damage to my throat. I wake up in the middle of the night sometimes coughing with liquid running down my throat. Trying to swallow my traditional meat is hard, and I do live alone.

Everything seems to be fine now, so I'm not scared. It's been over four years. I did my test recently and I'm still cancer free. I was supposed to do a test one July and they missed it, and that was hard. It scared me to miss an appointment and wait a whole year but then I got a phone call saying everything was fine. I'm grateful.

I went through a depression. I'm on medication for it. For many reasons, not just cancer. My life was torn apart. The business was down, I wasn't making money, my family was broken, then I got cancer, then COVID came, and then I was homeless. What else was going to be thrown at me? You can't take me from this earth because I have children. There's no way you're going to take them from me.

Medical travel sent my sister was with me as an escort sent when I went for surgery. I was in the hospital for about eleven days after the surgery because they had a tube in me and were draining liquids. It was really uncomfortable having that tube in me. My grandfather died of prostate cancer.

I stopped everything. I quit drinking and smoking cigarettes. I only drink tea; I don't drink coffee. I don't take salt anymore because my kidneys are running at a low percentage. The normal is 60–100 percent. I can quit anything. I've done that so many times in my life. I've had such an up and down life since my childhood. I was homeless at age 13. I did get myself through school. I did college, a couple years of mechanics. I worked for Kennicott Canada exploring the tundra for diamonds and we were the surveyors who found what is now Diavik Diamond Mine.[1] I can't work for anyone anymore because of the loss of part of my lung and I suffered a major concussion in 2017. It's messed up my memory and my balance is a little off, plus my hearing in my right ear is not great. I lost sight in my right eye as a child but I still have a perfect left eye. I can't go swinging a hammer, so I can't work for anybody. I am working on starting a new business and operating my own equipment. I prefer to work alone so I don't mind. I don't mind working at three in the morning until noon. Take the summers off and just travel with my children, enjoy the summer, then when they go back to school put myself back to work. That's my goal.

My daughter is 16 and my son is 11 years old, but I do have other children who are adults now. Cancer didn't really scare them because I explained that the cancer would be removed. It wasn't too stressful on them because the solution was provided by the doctor already. I didn't scare my children with thoughts of losing their father. That's one thing that scares me, leaving this world without being able to raise my children. I can't tell how the world will be when I'm gone so I'll do my best to ensure that I leave them with everything.

I was homeless at that time. Leaving Fort Simpson I had to take my business apart. I had to separate. I was in the process of moving back home and restarting over there. It's hard to start a business but as long as you have a plan, there's hope. That was my plan, but then COVID hit and then cancer hit. COVID really threw me off. My house wasn't liveable. The floor had collapsed and I couldn't live in it anymore, so they declared me homeless. They wouldn't work on my home either because I had to have lived in it for a year. But you can't live in it because it's unliveable and you can't fix it because you're not living in it. Like, what's wrong with you guys? I know it's a sturdy home. My grandfather built it. It's on a cement foundation. All the logs are upright. The roof has been changed but the floor is the one thing that needs fixing.

After I was out of lockdown for COVID, my sister found a place for me at Arnica Inn in Yellowknife.[2] I was at Arnica for eighteen months. Then I got a place with Housing First[3] and moved into an apartment. I don't have issues here. It's quiet. I have a good start. Business is hopefully going to start. I'm lucky. I ruined fifty years of my life to alcohol and drugs, not understanding what I was doing and the opportunities I had. I was the first one to be hired by Diavik. I quit because they gave me a hard hat and took my boat and fishing rod away from me. I walked away and moved to Fort Simpson and started my business.

I'm going to start up a business again. I'm going to buy myself a new truck. I'm looking forward to the future. I still have my hair. I didn't have to go through chemo. I was lucky to walk away. When I heard about lung cancer I thought, I'm done. I never heard of anyone surviving lung cancer. I know a few people, friends who had breast cancer, and I know what they went through and what happened to their bodies. So being able to walk away from it, I feel that my friends and family who have died are watching over me.

I've been through so many incidents in my life where I should have been gone. I shouldn't be here. I've dodged so many bullets in my life. I used to do hard drugs when I was young, and all those people I used to do drugs with are on the streets still, but I had support from my family. They were a phone call away and I could walk away from it. I was always able to quit. I was always tough that way. I quit for my children. I had a commitment to them. For me quitting is very easy.

I put so much in my lungs. Even living in the older houses, with their asbestos and lead, then crack cocaine, marijuana, and cigarettes. I put a lot of crap in my lungs. We used to hot knife when I was younger, and now I know we were inhaling metal. That's why I'm surprised I'm still here. Being raised and going through what I went through wasn't by choice.

Cancer motivated me. I've always had a plan, but I've always had obstacles too. Alcohol was the main obstacle. Cancer put me on alert. This is my last fifty years. I did the first fifty, I got another fifty to go. I will be a success. I will help people. I want to help people who are homeless on the streets, because I've been out there many times. I know what it's like to not have anything. To just need five bucks to eat. I try to help but addictions are hard to get rid of. If a friend of mine came up to me and told me they had terminal cancer, I wouldn't know how to handle it. A lady back home had the exact same thing I had, but she didn't go to the doctor, and they buried her a few months ago. That's where I would be too if I didn't go to the doctor. It did scare me, but there's no way I was going to let it beat me. She should have been here too, if she had gone in. If I had waited a year I would be where she is now.

Notes

1. Diavik Diamond Mine was the second diamond mine to begin operations in the Northwest Territories in 2002. It is located about 300 km Northeast of Yellowknife and depends on workers to fly in and fly out on shifts.
2. Starting in 2020, the former Arnica Inn was used as an isolation centre for around twenty-five people experiencing homelessness who were at high risk of complications stemming from COVID-19. The facility is now called Spruce Bough and provides permanent supportive housing and the territory's only Managed Alcohol Program. It is run by the Yellowknife Women's Society.
3. The Yellowknife Housing First Program supports chronically homeless adult individuals to access, maintain, and retain private market housing, providing a number of supports to assist participants to transition into housing and access the services they need. It is run by the Yellowknife Women's Society.

Lianne Mantla-Look

BEHCHOKǪ̀

I'm a registered nurse from the Tłı̨chǫ community of Behchokǫ̀, Northwest Territories. I live in Yellowknife with my husband, our beautiful daughter, and our two cats. I'm a stomach cancer survivor and this is my story.

As a registered nurse, I've been present with patients and their family members when a cancer diagnosis is received. I've had the privilege of providing care to patients with cancer and supporting their families during this incredibly tough journey. This experience prepared me for when my eldest sister was diagnosed with pancreatic cancer. She died when she was 38 years old, only a few months after her diagnosis.

Then I received my own cancer diagnosis when I was 34. I was diagnosed with stomach cancer after a routine gastroscopy in July 2015. After several biopsies to verify the location of the cancer in August, I had my stomach and surrounding lymph nodes removed in September of that same year.

The administrative frustration of my cancer diagnosis began the day I was told I had cancer. My husband and I were in Edmonton when the gastroenterologist called me with the news that changed our lives. It was fortuitous that we were in Edmonton because the gastroenterologist had discussed my case with the surgeon, and we were able to see him that morning.

Photo by Tessa Macintosh Photography.

Prior to meeting the surgeon for the first time, medical travel called me and informed me that we would not qualify for this benefit because my husband and I were technically on vacation when my surgical referral was arranged. It was suggested that, In order to qualify for my employment medical benefits, we fly home to Yellowknife and then fly back to Edmonton on another day to attend my appointment. This would have resulted in a delay in my surgery consult and overall medical care and testing. None of this made sense. There was no question; we were going to stay in Edmonton and deal with the fallout of medical travel later. I did not anticipate such administrative complications on top of a devastating diagnosis.

Once the consult was over, the plan was set, and I was booked in for surgery.

It was not an easy surgery. The procedure took approximately ten hours in the operating room and the recovery took several months. Afterwards I had to learn to live life without a stomach.

I was very clinical in my approach to how to handle my diagnosis. This was the only way I could cope with relinquishing my caregiver role and becoming a patient. I discussed my case daily with my surgical team, and my surgeon was receptive to questions I had. I had no concerns about the care I received from him and knew I was in good hands. I think my mom was surprised when I refused to act like a patient. She told me once that I was being disrespectful when I called my surgeon by his first name, but he actually would laugh at how informal we were being with each other. I mean, the man reconstructed my entire digestive system; he literally knew me inside and out.

My relationship with my husband changed significantly. I relied on him heavily as my caregiver and advocate. I was not used to being reliant on someone for all my daily needs and I hated feeling so helpless, but I was grateful for the incredible support he provided. As my caregiver, my husband was given a crash course in post-operative care, wound care, and pain management. He spoke on my behalf to the nurses when I was unable to. He was there when the surgeons began their rounds at 6:30 every morning, and he didn't leave my side until I was given my last medication of the day at 10:00 each night. Whenever I had an emergency situation during the night, he was back in the hospital within minutes. He was a major factor in my recovery. I know I would not have done as well if I hadn't had him by my side.

Before my diagnosis, I had no idea you could live life without an essential organ such as a stomach. My new diet was trial and error, and it took me time to get used to a stomach-less life. I had to eat every two to three hours otherwise my blood glucose levels would drop. I also couldn't eat and drink fluid at the same time because this moved food into my digestive system too quickly. I was only able to drink fluids before I ate, which resulted in not having enough room for food, or I had to wait an hour after eating to drink fluids and by that time it I had to eat again. It was exhausting.

This new eating schedule made other aspects of my life challenging. Simple things like running errands required planning around my food intake. I had to have a snack before I left the house, and I couldn't be gone for more than an hour before I had to rush home to have another snack or meal. I found it tough to make plans with friends at restaurants because I couldn't rely on my ordered food to be prepared in a timely manner. It took me months before I could make the hour-long drive to see my mother in Behchokǫ̀ because I had to plan my meals around the trip.

It's easy to assume that I could have just packed food for my outings, but I was still learning how to eat after having my stomach removed, and all food items and food groups were trial and error for the first year. Whatever was okay the previous day wasn't necessarily okay to eat the next day, and the wrong food at the wrong time would make me violently ill. If I was going to be sick, I preferred to be in the comfort of my own home rather than out in public.

I was on disability leave from work, and the disability insurance representative who was assigned to me called six months after my surgery to ask if I was going back to work soon. I informed them that my surgeon recommended a year off to recover in case I had any complications. The representative said that they had Google searched the recovery timeline for stomach cancer and according to the internet I should be ready to go back to work six months post-op. I firmly reminded them I was going to be following my doctor's recommendations to be off work for the full year. I also reminded the representative that I was approved to be on disability for a year. Not much was said beyond that until I was ready to transition back to work and provided my employer and the disability representative with a progress update. Sometimes it felt like a full-time job just dealing with the administrative side of being sick and recovering. While I appreciated my medical travel and other benefits, navigating these administrative processes was so challenging.

I was off work for a year after my surgery and then slowly transitioned back to nursing. I had to leave my position as a community health nurse because I couldn't commute for two hours a day with my new eating schedule. I started a new position that was closer to home, which was better for me in terms of distance and the pace of work.

I also faced other health issues. One afternoon during my second month at my new job, I developed a cough and fever at work. After a week where I went to the ER twice and saw my family doctor twice and was told I had the flu, I eventually got a chest x-ray that revealed I had pneumonia and was admitted to hospital for a week. A few months later, I began to have abdominal pain after work. The pain intensified and then I began to vomit. Do you have any idea how painful it is to vomit with no stomach? I called my primary physician, and he advised me to go to the ER right away. I had to have a CT and was told I had gallstones and would need to be admitted for observation. I declined the hospital admission because I didn't want to be in the hospital again. I assured the ER doctor that I could manage the pain at home and would return to the ER if I needed to. A couple of days later I was informed I would need my gallbladder removed.

I was determined to have this procedure done in Edmonton by the surgeon who removed my stomach. I trusted him completely and I simply did not want another surgeon who didn't know me or was unaware of my surgical history to perform this new surgery. My experience as a health-care provider and my knowledge of the Northern health and medical travel systems helped me advocate for myself. Without this background, I don't think I could have been as successful at advocating for my needs, and I worry about those patients who don't have the familiarity to self-advocate in the same way.

I sent all my lab tests and imaging results to my surgeon in Edmonton, and we set a date for the removal of my gallbladder. The only obstacle I encountered was that I did not have a referral for my surgery to be performed out of territory. I saw a locum doctor because my family doctor was away. The locum was adamant that I did not require this procedure outside of Yellowknife. It wasn't until I provided my rationale for the surgery and a detailed account of my total gastrectomy that the locum doctor agreed with me. They actually admitted that they did not read my chart in full and were ready to deny me the referral before they saw me, based on the fact that this type of routine surgery was one that could be performed in Yellowknife. They had no idea that I had already arranged the procedure; I just needed the referral to get the medical travel process started. Again, I was surprised by the amount of administration involved in being sick, recovering, and just accessing the care for myself that I knew I needed and that I knew could best support me to get back on my feet.

Although I did not have any further significant medical setbacks following my second surgery, I continue to have challenges with respect to my diet to this day. Some days food is not for enjoyment but for fuel and energy, and sometimes I find it tedious to need to eat so often. I still plan my outings around my eating schedule, I never leave the house without a granola bar or fruit, and I have glucose pills in all my bags and in both of our vehicles. I'm considered cured by my surgeon and gastroenterologist, and for this reason I tend not to worry about the possibility of recurrence.

When I reflect on that time, I think the most frustrating part of my cancer experience was the administrative aspect of receiving a life-changing diagnosis like cancer and having to worry about how you're going to get home from another province. I realize that I was more fortunate than most people in my situation. For example, we were not set back financially by choosing to remain in Edmonton that day at the very beginning of my diagnosis. However, administrative challenges were present at every stage of my cancer experience.

I hope that people working on the caregiving and administrative side of the health system can read my story and gain some insight into what it's like to be a patient. It is important that they know how much weight their words and actions carry for patients. For those at the start of a cancer diagnosis, I hope my story can help prepare them for what is ahead and let them know they have the right to ask for what they need and deserve.

I don't think about my cancer experience every moment of the day anymore, but it's never far from my mind. It's changed me as a nurse and as a person; it's made me more of an advocate for patients. It also reminds me to focus on living my life. When I found out I was pregnant, I called my surgeon to give him the incredible news. He was genuinely happy for me and wished me the best. The last time I spoke to him was to inform him that I gave birth to a beautiful baby girl, and his last message was, "Enjoy your baby." And that's what I'm going to do.

Cecilia Rabesca

BEHCHOKÒ

I'm 58 years of age, and I was born and raised in Behchokǫ̀, Northwest Territories. My late parents are Adele Marie and Jimmy Rabesca, and thankfully they have not witnessed my illness. I have eight living siblings and lost two and others before I was born. I was raised a Catholic and remain a believer of Jesus Christ our Lord to this day. But I know that everyone has their own beliefs; it's a personal choice and I respect that.

In the summer of 2017 on a beautiful Saturday morning, while I was taking a shower, I decided to do my monthly well-woman's check and found a lump. Naturally, it was a shock. It felt like a bucket of cold water was thrown at me.

Prior to this, I had many lumps, but they always turned out to be benign, meaning they were not cancerous. Nonetheless, whenever I would find a lump, it was always a shock. I went through many thoughts, "What should I do? Where do I go? Can this be seen quickly? What if I don't have a regular doctor? What's going to happen to me and my family? I hope it's not cancer." So many thoughts and questions.

Through my ordeal of getting this one particular lump checked, I often heard the words, "You're a very lucky lady." We only have a visiting doctor in the community on Wednesdays, and I found this lump on a Saturday morning. My mind was racing. I thought

Photo provided by Tłı̨chǫ Government.

of going to the hospital emergency room in Yellowknife, but I wasn't sure if it was an emergency — I mean, it wasn't like I was having a heart attack. So, I stayed home and did my regular routine and other mindless activities to keep from over thinking.

Then on Sunday evening I got a message on my phone saying a family member was at our local clinic because of a health scare, and I joined them to keep them company. It turns out it was okay. As I was sitting with them, a nurse came in and said, "If anyone has any questions, I'll be at my desk for the next 15 minutes." I thought it was a good opportunity to speak to the nurse. She gave me advice about the lump and told me to book an appointment the next day. I phoned the clinic in Yellowknife early the next morning to get an appointment. After that initial appointment the doctors fast-tracked my next appointments, including getting in to see a surgeon from Edmonton who happened to be at the Stanton Hospital with another surgeon. It turns out they had time to fit me in. They told me I was a lucky lady. They did a biopsy and sent it to Edmonton, and the results did not turn out well.

It was during the time that I planned to go to Lac Ste. Anne for a week's pilgrimage[1] that I got a call saying I needed to go to Edmonton for another biopsy. Once home, I got a call from the surgeon that I had seen in Yellowknife. He told me that the lump was positive. I left the appointment feeling numb. My tears wanted to burst like a dam, but I was in a hospital full of people in the waiting area. I just stood there. Then I saw a friend who worked at the hospital. She just happened to be walking by. When she saw me, I must've been as white as a ghost because she grabbed me and asked, "What's wrong?" I looked at her without words and she guided me towards the washroom quickly and said, "I'll watch the door." The dam of tears burst, and I cried for what seemed like a long time. When I finally stopped crying, I was very thankful for that friend to be in the right place at the right time.

The next thing I had to do was inform my family members and community. It was hard to do, but it was the right thing to do. Through tears they were informed. Most everyone prayed for a good outcome. My favourite person made me some on-the-land medicine and taught about traditional medicine, which I'm thankful for to this day.

On Sundays I usually help the local priest at church, which I have done for years and still do. Nothing was going to stop me from the volunteer work I did with the church. My church family needed to know that changes were going to start happening to my body, as I had opted to do all treatments. My favourite person stood beside me and encouraged me to be strong as I shared the news. In tears again, I told the congregation I had been diagnosed with cancer and I was to undergo surgery and treatment. The positive feedback and prayers were amazing, and over time, others who had cancer came forward too and shared some of their own stories. The amount of people who have cancer in our communities is a big eye opener. I hope to continue working with them.

Next thing I knew I was assigned a triage nurse, who monitored me while I went through the process of dealing with all the doctors and appointments. I went to Edmonton and my spouse came with me for support. I saw a surgeon who advised me to have the lump removed as soon as possible because they can grow fast. By then it had been two months since my initial discovery of the lump.

In the fall, I took time off work. I was not sure when I would be back to work. I got scheduled for surgery in Edmonton. Before the surgery I had to make the decision on whether to cut out the lump only, cut out my entire breast or take half of my breast out. I have never been so conflicted in my life. The decision was only mine to make. In the end I opted to get just the lump removed. As a woman, these parts of you are very important and to lose or alter them is something very personal.

The surgeon came to see me right before I was taken into the operating room and asked, "Is there anything you want to ask of me before you are wheeled in?" I said to him, "Take only what needs to be taken out." He held my hand and looked at me directly and said, "Yes." He was the first person I saw upon waking up and he said again, "You're a lucky lady! We took out the small lump which was encased in a ball of fat." He left and I never saw him again. He was a wonderful surgeon, but I do hope to never see him again in my lifetime.

About two months later I recovered and was set up for chemo, which was done in Yellowknife. It was heart wrenching for me to do chemo because I knew it was a poison that is put in your bloodstream to attack the cancer. My first two days taking chemo were okay but on the third day I found myself sitting up at three in the morning. I couldn't sleep. My whole body felt weird. My nights turned into day and my days turned into night. I had waves of nausea. I couldn't eat, I couldn't sleep,

I was constipated. Delivering a baby was easier than being constipated after each chemo treatment. Never mind the colour!! My menopause kicked in and went into overdrive. Two weeks after the first chemo I was in the shower washing my hair and some of my hair stayed in my hand. It was shocking, but I knew this would happen eventually. They tell you about hair loss, but nothing can really prepare you for that. I gently washed the shampoo out for fear of losing all of my hair right then and there. I kept finding hair everywhere. It was discouraging so I did what I was advised to do by a wonderful Elder in my life: I shaved my head after my family left for work. I sat on the floor in front of the wood stove, which was firing away. First, I brushed my hair out thinking I could brush everything out but that was impossible, so I took my spouse's shaver and shaved every hair on my head as tears ran down my face. I instantly felt a draft. I looked at the mound of hair and offered it to the fire while praying for speedy healing. I put on the toque that the Cross Cancer Institute had given me and continued crying up a storm for the loss of my hair. I ended up getting a wig. I had a few and they kept my head warm. Even now talking about it is very hard. It is a sad memory, and I feel for those who are going through this ordeal now.

My body went through so many different changes including waking up in the middle of the night thinking I was paralyzed. I couldn't move. My back was in excruciating pain, but they tell you not to take any pain medications in case over-the-counter drugs have a reaction with the chemo.

I went on disability even though I was encouraged to go back to work right away. It would be really hard to go back to work because of the side effects of the chemo. I was so discouraged. At the same time, I was lucky to be getting disability benefits because I had bills to pay.

I was offered a clinical trial called Neulasta in pill form. I was told it would help with my nausea so I agreed, and thank God it was covered by my benefits from work. I felt very lucky because it was costly just for one small vial. The nurses in my community taught me how to self-administer it into the fat of my tummy. It was quick and painless. For someone who does not like needles, I sure had to have a lot of needles. My poor veins, they held up through constant blood work, chemo, Neulasta, and more.

Once my chemo was done, a few months were given to allow my body to rest before I had to start radiation. Radiation was done in

Edmonton at the Cross Cancer Institute. I had to do twenty rounds from Monday to Friday. They started at 11:45 am daily and took less than five minutes. It did not hurt. I was put in a hotel room paid for by my spouse's benefits. I was happy that I got to spend some time on my own. Other patients are put up at Larga, where there are conveniences, but I was happy to be on my own because I got to reflect a lot on how I should treat myself better.

When I got home, two weeks later, I felt the effects of the radiation to a point where even a piece of clothing couldn't touch the area where my skin was radiated. My skin was inflamed. All I could do was wait for it to go away and put ointment on. I went back to the Cross Cancer Institute for a final check-up and brought back a wig I had signed out. I was given a prescription for hormone pills to take daily for five years. I was informed that the type of cancer I had made my hormones attack my body so the pill they gave me would help, but it didn't do much for my menopause. That day when I left the Cross Cancer Institute for the last time, I stood outside the big doors and prayed with tears asking God to please never bring me back to that place again. I prayed for everyone affected by cancer. My hair eventually came back greyish black. I tell people to this day that I got burnt inside out and it affected my hair.

In being diagnosed with cancer, family became even more important. I got help from naturopathic doctors, which I didn't hide from the regular doctors. I took vitamins and figured out which ones I could take with chemo and radiation and which ones I could not, including what foods to eat and not to eat with each treatment. The vitamins helped with pain and kept my bones and body strong.

I saw a small black-like snake travel quickly in my veins one day and it shook me to my core. But now I am back at work from 9–5 daily. My life is busy. I still have high hopes of helping other cancer patients in my community as I didn't know where to go when I first found out I had the big C. It would've been nice to have someone to chat with for advice on what to do. I do that for those that come up to me now in confidence and pray for them to be strong. Masì.

Note

1   Each summer, many Indigenous Catholics from across Western and Northern Canada travel on an annual pilgrimage to a spiritual gathering at Lac Ste. Anne, west of Edmonton.

Florence Barnaby

FORT GOOD HOPE

I'm from Fort Good Hope, and I'm 79 years old. Our community has been hit hard with cancer. We now have cancer screening in place for residents every two years. We blame it on the pollution coming downstream from the South into the Mackenzie River.

I went to Inuvik for a colonoscopy. They said nothing was wrong with me. Later on, I travelled to Ottawa for a meeting about cancer. There, I learned about a First Nations reserve where the lakes and land have no pollution, but they have still been hit hard with cancer. After returning from this meeting, I requested another colonoscopy and gastroscopy. It was then that the cancer was found. It was a good thing I requested testing again.

It was while I was home in Fort Good Hope that I received the phone call stating I had cancer. I was shocked. I thought I had looked after my health. At the time, I was in a local cancer support group called Goba, facilitated by Melinda Laboucan. I went to various events organized by Melinda, who later founded Goba Care in Edmonton.

After my diagnosis, I travelled to Yellowknife for medical. While I was there it really hit me that I had cancer. I began having thoughts like, "Why me?" It was really hard to take in. I was walking down the streets

Photo by Alexa Scully.

of Yellowknife, crying! Good thing that I knew some counsellors there in Yellowknife. So, I went and spent two hours or so with my counsellor. I tried to accept my diagnosis of cancer, but I couldn't believe it. I didn't know what kind of cancer I had either. I didn't have any symptoms. I was already at that time living a healthy lifestyle. I thought, "How am I going to live my life to survive this?" I experienced a lot in the beginning, but disbelief was the biggest challenge for me.

My husband was the first person I told when I was diagnosed. Then I told my sisters. It seemed like none of them believed me. They looked at me and asked, "You?" We have seen people on their deathbed from cancer, but it looked like nothing was wrong with me physically. I told some friends too, but it was very hard to tell my kids. It's very hard to have to tell your family that you've been diagnosed with cancer. Very few of the people I knew who had cancer survived. I have grandchildren and to have to tell them was really hard. I had to make lots of phone calls to them. It was not an easy thing to do; it was hard on everyone.

What really helped me during that time was the community's cancer support group. We met and formed a sharing circle. We spoke about what we were going through with cancer, and I didn't feel alone because other group members were going through the same thing. We would share our feelings, our worries, our stress, and other issues. I really enjoyed the sharing circle. We met twice a month. Other events in the community helped too.

For example, during cancer week in June, we planned a community walk for cancer with Melinda Laboucan and Goba Care. All the kids in the community joined in, and we made a big circle on the banks of the Mackenzie River. We exercised twice a week at the school. Melinda planned a lot of activities along with sharing circles. She did home visits with cancer patients. She would sit and have tea with me, too. I would share about cancer, and I would share my personal life struggles too, like my worries about my children. I really tried to stay away from stress. I have been able to go back into the healing work I was doing before I got cancer. I had been working on my healing journey from the harms of residential school. I really got good at dealing with what I was going through now and in the past.

We went berry picking as a group. Melinda would harvest berries and distribute berries to the group for those who couldn't come out on the land with us. Being out on the land is really beneficial when dealing with stress. I have my cabin, and I go there sometimes too. We also went out for traditional medicine and got spruce gum and various other medicinal plants. Melinda would go on our local radio station and give out information about cancer too. As a group we also created a little booklet on self-care and healthy lifestyles.

All these group activities were good, but sadly they shut down when Melinda moved away from Fort Good Hope. I gave her a call and told her I'd like to restart our group again. It's so important that people are not alone and to know that there are others who are going through the same thing. Since Melinda moved away, I've been thinking of restarting our group. It is something to look forward to. Sharing circles are helpful. I think we should have a cancer support group in every community across the North.

There are a lot of people who have cancer who are worse off than others. Some people are told they have maybe a month or a year or less to live. My sister died of cancer. It was hard on me. Her death could have been prevented by early cancer screening but that didn't happen for her. You go through a questioning stage, asking "Why?" It's so hard to deal with; I still get very emotional.

Sharing circles really helped. I also have a Christian group called Phone-a-Friend. I'm thankful for them. I can just pick up the phone and talk and share anything about what I'm dealing with, and it is anonymous and confidential. I had friends in the community that I phone to talk to as well. I had a very close friend who died a year ago, Alphonsine McNeely. I always phoned her. I have pictures of her. In every picture of her, she's always laughing. In the times when I feel down and like no one cares, I make phone calls to people. I would often call Alphonsine. It didn't matter what time, day or night; she was always laughing. I still think of her when I feel down. It's always good to have a friend to visit and laugh with.

Visits from community members are helpful too. It's really hard to face cancer alone, but it's easier if you have friends. I have a family, and I have a husband who looks after me. Some days when I don't feel well it's nice knowing he's there to look after me. I think I got spoiled from cancer! I have a son who is always there asking me, "Mom, how are you doing?" All my kids check on me. I have two daughters who live in Edmonton. They phone me all the time. Family support is important. Knowing that I am not alone is good.

What motivates me to keep going even though I have cancer is that I don't want to die. I still have goals to conquer. I've always been active in reviving our language and culture. We cannot separate the two. I want to continue to promote our language. We were a strong nation at one time. I always think, "How do we preserve our culture?" I have lots of plans. I retired from my job as the community alcohol and drug counsellor. I was there for many years, and I regret retiring early. I used to travel to all the communities. We have a problem in our communities with new drugs coming out on the street. We've lost a lot of people from alcohol- and drug-related deaths in our communities. I ask myself, "How can I make a better future for my grandchildren?" You can't just expect it to get better without putting in the work. We have to talk about it. We have to make plans and offer programs to make our community a healthy place to live.

That's been my goal ever since I became an Elder. I don't want my grandchildren to go through what I went through. I got into alcohol when I was in my twenties. I don't want that for my family. I want others to know that there's hope! Getting sober is the best thing I ever did. Now I'm happy even though I have cancer. I'm not dwelling on cancer. I'm eventually going to die either way, but I want to accomplish something before I go. I may die from old age, I don't know.

Once we are strong in our culture, we will be a strong nation again. When I was growing up there used to be drum dances and hand games when we would come into the community. I was 10 years old when I first saw someone highly intoxicated. It's not good for little children to see that. I wonder what kind of future kids today are going to have. When I was growing up, my friends and I had fun and we never had to drink to be happy. There's hope. I want to see my community happy and healthy again. That is my goal.

I think cancer happened to me for a reason. It really woke me up. I used to think that I was healthy but when I found out I had cancer I changed my lifestyle even more. When I sobered up, I thought I was healthy. I started eating vegetables. I was stress free. I was going to counselling. Counselling helped me to not dwell on the past. I'm not thankful for the cancer, but it made me do something to deal with the other issues that I was carrying.

I encourage everyone to get screened for cancer especially if it runs in your family. Some people get screened every four to ten years, but that's too long to wait for testing. Go sooner; it's available. If I had waited four more years as I had planned, the cancer could have advanced. You can't blame the health department; it's up to us to live healthy. I haven't smoked for thirty-two years, and it's been thirty-three years since I had a drink. I eat vegetables, not junk food. You can live a good life if you practise prevention.

When I was first told that I had a lump in my stomach, they wanted to cut it out, but they didn't and it grew bigger. So, I went to Edmonton for chemotherapy and radiation. I was okay during the treatment but a month or so after I got home, I couldn't eat, and I was losing weight. I didn't understand what was going on. Post-treatment symptoms and side effects weren't explained when they should have been. This caused me stress and I wanted to give up. I thought, "What's the use?" Then those symptoms passed, and I began eating again. I was told that these were the side effects of radiation therapy. Even today, sometimes I'll be talking and then all of a sudden, I will forget what I was talking about. I had some friends explain that brain fog is a side effect of radiation too. I was never told about it by the doctors.

I still have to go through tests, and I just recently had a biopsy during my colonoscopy procedure. I always fear the doctors telling me that the cancer has gotten worse. I have friends that were told during their check-ups that their cancer increased to stage 4 and they were given a short life expectancy. That's what I'm afraid to hear, that my cancer has advanced. Right now, I'm going through tests, and these thoughts are crossing my mind. I have a very good escort who knows and understands me. Mabel Kakfwi is always there to help me, not because I'm old but because she wants to be there for me. I have had different friends come with me to Edmonton on medical travel and sometimes my husband comes with me too. Medical escorts are so helpful. But you can't just grab someone off the street to come with you; it has to be somebody you know. You have to have someone accompany you who understands you and is able to talk to you. It is very helpful for me to have friends who care who can be my escort.

At first, the doctors didn't tell me what type of cancer I had. This caused me a lot of stress. I know friends who were told they had kidney, liver, or lung cancer. That was the worst thing for me. Later, when I was told what type of cancer I had, I Googled it and found out it was not an aggressive type. I felt the doctor should have told me what type of cancer it was when he first told me I had cancer. That would have been so beneficial to know back then.

The type of cancer I have is not aggressive. I nicknamed my cancer "Lazy Joe" because it's lazy. My cancer is called lymphoma. This type of cancer is found in the lymph nodes but it was discovered by the colonoscopy I requested. I don't know how they found it through a colonoscopy because I have lumps in my neck area. I have a lump in my lower abdomen too. I do self-examinations for any new lumps, and I still go to Cross Cancer for check-ups. I have a really nice doctor who even phones me at home to see how I'm doing. He's a good friend who cares. When I tell friends of these phone calls, they say, "My doctor never phones me!" My experience at Cross Cancer in Edmonton was very positive.

My family and I are more aware of cancer now that I have been diagnosed. It's good to let your family know. I have always been close to my family, but cancer brings you closer together. When you're first diagnosed you have thoughts like, "Will I have time to spend with my grandkids?" I am especially close to my grandkids. My granddaughter Chanelle is so happy when she sees me.

I was diagnosed around five years ago. Ever since I retired, I've been writing in my spare time. Writing helps with my memory. I've been writing and collecting stories from Elders. I feel okay, and I always say I'm okay too. Your mind plays a big role in your well-being. Keep in mind that you control cancer, cancer does not control you! I wasn't going to let it. I'm strong! I'm tough!

Over the years, I've been approached by people who have been diagnosed with cancer. I welcome them to talk to me and I let them know that they are not alone. I let them know I'm here to listen. I always say there's hope and we can beat it. When I was first diagnosed, I needed someone to talk to about it. I went to a counsellor right away. I'm here to help because I went through same thing. I know what helped me through that experience. It's always good to be a listener to someone who needs it. It helps you too when you help others. Helping others makes you feel needed and trusted, which makes you feel good too.

~

In memory of Florence Barnaby: January 14, 1942, to October 7, 2024

Melinda Laboucan

FORT GOOD HOPE

My maiden last name is Grandjambe. I am married to Gregory Laboucan from Whitefish Lake, Alberta. I'm originally from Fort Good Hope, Northwest Territories. I am K'asho Got'ine. My mother is the late Janet Grandjambe. She passed away in September 2011 from cancer. My father is Anthony Grandjambe. My father's parents are Michel and Rosie Grandjambe. My mother's parents are Denise and Thomas Manuel.

I pretty much lived in and around Fort Good Hope my entire life. My dad used to go trapping. In the early years of my life, we lived three hours down from Fort Good Hope in a place we call Little Chicago. From September to December my dad would bring all of us down there with my auntie Angela and my uncle Joe Grandjambe. It was there we learned the basics of living out on the land — watching my granny Rosie and my essa Michel; they did things traditionally. I used to watch my granny work on traditional medicine from the land. I always knew that one day I would also use it.

My journey was tough growing up as I am the oldest of four siblings. Like so many in my community and across the North, we are part of the intergenerational trauma of residential school and its impacts. To this day, I don't blame my parents. I love and have so much respect for my parents, but growing up with them was tough. We had to make a lot of amends while they were on earth. Even though my dad didn't talk about his feelings, I know he loved me.

Later in my twenties my mother and I became close and experienced deep grace and forgiveness. I was able to take advantage of many opportunities because of my mother who got me there. The one that had the biggest impact on my life was my mother helping me get into John Paul II Bible School in Radway, Alberta. This led to a ministry that involved working with six senior citizen residences in Edmonton, St. Albert, and Legal, Alberta. This was followed by an opportunity to move to Edmonton to work with the homeless community and gave me a real love for the city of Edmonton and its people.

My mom was such a huge part of our family and the wider community. Everybody flocked to her. Her heart truly shone on the outside. My mom was joyful and welcoming. She would invite visitors to Fort Good Hope over to her house and she would cook for them. My mom was that light that everybody went to. She was there for people who were struggling with their addiction and mental health issues. She was so gifted in her sewing and beadwork, and she loved to share her skills.

In 2009, my mother was sent from Fort Good Hope to isolation in Yellowknife with suspected tuberculosis. When the TB test came back negative she was released from hospital and sent home. They sent her for another test in Inuvik as they wanted to know more about the spot on my mother's lungs. But the test in Inuvik did not give any results. From that point, we received no further follow-up.

By June 2011 my mother could not walk. The nurse in Fort Good Hope was rude and forced her to get up and walk. My mother felt disrespected and made to feel she was lying about the level of pain she was in. Not too long after, she was medevacked to Inuvik. We didn't know what was wrong, but we didn't suspect it was cancer because no one else in my family had it and my mom was so young. My mom was trying to be strong for us but deep down she was afraid and alone.

When the doctors in Inuvik still couldn't figure out what was wrong, they sent my mom to Edmonton. Immediately my family gathered and raised funds to get my father and me to Edmonton to be with her. Test after test was done. My mom's doctor and Northern Health Services Network[1] came into the hospital room and sat us down and they told us the news that shattered our entire lives: my mom had cancer.

When my mother was diagnosed there was no one in Edmonton who could explain to us what was happening in a way we could hear and really understand. The doctors gave us the clinical update and left. No one showed us how to prepare for the next few months. Looking back, we needed someone who knew where we were coming from to tell us what to expect when someone has end-stage cancer and wants to go back home to their remote community for their final days. We had to figure everything out on our own, in our shock and devastation.

Thankfully the communities across the Sahtu and Delta came together to fundraise again. More family were able to come to Edmonton to be with us and our mother. This is just one thing I love about my home and how our Northern communities pull together in hard times. I miss that in the big city where you just don't see it.

We had to wait for a medevac plane to come to Edmonton from the NWT to bring my mom back home. My dad got onto the medevac with my mom and together they flew to Inuvik. The rest of us, all twelve of us, got on the plane and flew back to Yellowknife and then Fort Good Hope. We rested one day before getting on a boat for eleven hours to travel down the Mackenzie River to Inuvik. We needed to be with Mom. When we got to Tsiighetchic there were trucks there waiting for us. It was late, but they knew the urgency and they drove us the rest of the way to Inuvik. The people of Inuvik got us a hotel and everything we needed. People were cooking for us and dropping off food. We were overwhelmed by the love and support. That's what I always hold close to me. When we were going through the worst thing on earth, the people of Inuvik showed us love, and that lifted us up and helped us keep going.

We were in Inuvik for about a week. When it was time to go back to Fort Good Hope my mom wanted me to get on the plane with her. When we were leaving Inuvik, a nurse came up to me and pulled me aside. She gave me two bags of medicine and told me they were for pain management for my mom. She told me how to administer it. My eyes were big, and fear set in. I asked, "Aren't the nurses going to be there to help us?" The answer was, "We don't know." We just had to figure it all out once we got there. I had no idea what it was going to be like when we got back to Fort Good Hope, but for the three weeks my mom was still with us, our house was filled with people. People were sleeping everywhere, even on the floor. We had a fire going outside every single day. People were even flying in to be with my mom.

To be a caregiver at the end of life is an honour and privilege. It is also a deeply painful experience that you will have to live with until your journey is done on earth. You need to learn to find healthy ways to cope when you are triggered by the things you experience as a caregiver. My mom only wanted my auntie and me to provide her care, including administering the pain medications and helping her eat and wash. No one told us about things like shifting her from side to side so that she would not suffer with bed sores. The nurses came in but just to check vital signs. We were left alone with very little support at every stage. We had to learn fast while being brave, comforting, and calm. Every day we prayed together for our strong mother to be healed but it was her time. The hardest part was accepting our last talk with her that she is tired and can't fight anymore. How do you even let go of the one person on this earth who was there every step of the way? She was our comfort, our security, our supporter. I still miss her hugs and comforting voice.

My father died 13 months and 11 days after my mom passed. Life was just too hard for him without Mom. My siblings and I became orphans, and we had to learn fast to do life without our parents. My sister Ryanna needed end-of-life care shortly after our parents died. She was our angel, she held our family together, she had a beautiful contagious smile that would light up any room. She had special needs that meant she couldn't talk or walk, but she had a way to make you feel loved. She loved Neil Diamond because Dad always listened to him. Ryanna was devastated when Mom and Dad passed away as she was very close to them. She ended up getting very sick. I knew that her time was coming to an end, and through many conversations with medical professionals and my family, we decided to bring Ryanna home to Fort Good Hope from Inuvik. Dr. Leah Seaman helped advocate for us to get the support we needed. Two nurses came to the house on rotation to provide end-of-life care. With my mom we didn't have time to fully be there with her because we were in constant caregiving mode. Because of the nursing support, we were given that time to just be there in Ryanna's presence, holding her, talking to her, and comforting her. We had the fire going every day outside and my uncles played the drum as she loved the drum. We had an enormous amount of support. That's what helps the most, a support system to keep you strong.

After this series of losses, I asked myself, "What can I do to help families like us?" I had a deep passion to help others through their grief. I worked many jobs in Fort Good Hope as a coordinator for youth, prenatal care, wellness and cancer care. I worked with the NWT Breast Cancer Action Group[2] to help with developing the cancer survivor care plan. The work was well received, and after one year, Yamoga Land Corporation[3] funded me for another year.

This was at a time when survivors didn't want to talk about cancer because the belief was if you talk too much about it, it will come back. We had to approach that belief with patience, love, and no judgement. We brought people together through food with no agenda. Then we added sharing circles. We needed to get the word out so we went on the local radio station to talk about what we were doing. Then we had Elders join us to talk about traditional medicine. We went out on the land and learned about harvesting medicine. I love the land. There's so much power and peace out there.

My drive to support cancer care was on fire! The people of Fort Good Hope wanted a name for this work, a name that was going to mean something to us and also bring hope to anyone newly diagnosed with cancer, survivors, and their families. The group working together in the community consisted of all the front-line workers in Fort Good Hope: cancer survivors, Elders, youth, the local store managers, leadership, the nurses, everybody and anybody that had a passion to support anyone going through cancer. Together as a group we found a name that meant something: Goba, which means "light on the horizon" in our Dene language. Goba was the first cancer support group operating in NWT.

Losing loved ones is hard. I still get triggered at times. When you lose someone close to you it is hard to want to be on this earth. We are not meant to be here forever. "We are just passing through" is something my mother often said to me.

I learned so many things through both my mom's and my sister's experience through end-of-life care. I learned how to advocate. I learned how to talk to health professionals and politicians to best support families in small remote communities across the North in their health-care journeys.

When I moved to Edmonton in 2018, I didn't want my work to end, and I launched Goba Care in October 2021. The work of Goba

Care comes out of my experience: we provide material support, advocacy, navigation, and cultural connection. We customize our care based on individual needs. At some point in the cancer journey, travel to Edmonton is almost always necessary. About a quarter of Goba Care clients are in Edmonton receiving cancer care. I know how hard medical travel can be. Here in Edmonton I can serve Northern patients and help Southern health-care providers improve the quality of care they offer to Northerners.

Before my mom was diagnosed I knew nothing about cancer. I've learned so much along the way. I wouldn't be here doing the work that I'm doing if it wasn't for the amount of support I received from family and community. You can't stand in this world by yourself. You need a community to surround you. I am truly grateful for my husband, children, grandchildren, my colleague Kate Kerber, and the amount of love and support that came from my late granny Denise Manuel and my amazing family and friends. Mahsi.

Notes

1. The Northern Health Services Network offers assistance to people from Yukon, Nunavut, and NWT who are referred to Edmonton for medical care. It is provided by Alberta Health Services.
2. The Breast Cancer Action Group is a non-profit society and charity that promotes breast health, fosters hope, and works to ease the journey of Northerners impacted by breast cancer and other cancers.
3. The Yamoga Land Corporation is a land-claim driven corporation that works to achieve social and economic self-sufficiency for Fort Good Hope participants of the Sahtu Dene and Metis Comprehensive Land Claim Agreement.

Grace Martin

FORT MCPHERSON

My parents are James and Edith Nerysoo. My grandparents from my mom's side are Ronnie and Laura Pascal, and from my dad's side are William and Catherine Nerysoo. I was born and raised in Fort McPherson. Growing up we spent our summers at a fish camp with my grandparents Ronnie and Laura. In the winter I stayed at the hostel to go to school. In the early seventies I came to Inuvik to go to high school. I quit high school because of alcohol in the home. I got married at a young age and had three children, Bella Kathy, Brenda, and Brian Dean, and adopted my youngest daughter, Brianna. I separated from my husband, who eventually passed away from alcohol. Alcohol was a big factor in my life until I had my first grandchild, which was when I made a decision to leave alcohol. It has made a big impact on the people I love. I have worked various camp jobs but now I stay home and sew.

When I came home from residential school, I was able to eat what I wanted and do what I wanted. I was able to run around free and do whatever I wanted. In the hostel, there was a big fence around it and if you ever went outside of the fence, you'd get punished — punished harshly too. There were so many rules. We went to church twice a day, and we had to kneel to pray, and if you turned around you got slapped in the head. If

---

Mary Effie Snowshoe and Grace Martin.

you didn't want food and turned it away, it was forced down your throat. I remember one time I didn't want spinach, and the supervisor shoved it down my throat to the point that I wanted to throw up. Today you look at kids and they are so free in school; they do what they want. But with us, we had to go by the rules of the missionaries. We were able to go home to our families three times a year: Easter, summer break, and Christmas holidays.

 I first learned what cancer was when my grandmother Catherine passed away from it. I was really young. I heard my dad telling someone she had stomach cancer. In middle school, my grandfather Ronnie passed away of cancer. Then my dad was diagnosed with colon cancer, so my siblings and I had to get tested. I kept putting my test off because I was scared to get tested. I finally went to get tested, but when I was ready to leave, they told me I couldn't. Then two doctors came into the room and diagnosed me with colon cancer.

 I was all alone in the room and the room went white. All I could see was the doctor's face and nothing else. I must have gone into some kind of shock. I started thinking, "I wonder how long I have to live and how far along it is." There was another person in the room beside me, Florence Furlong. She was there with me all that day and she showed her support. Then I had to think of how to tell my dad, who was in long-term care in Inuvik on his deathbed from the same cancer. We were both diagnosed around the same time. When my dad found out I had cancer too, I don't think he really understood as he was on palliative care by that time. It was so hard to tell him knowing I was going to lose him. I went to see him, and my sister Phyllis was there. I told her of my diagnosis and asked her, "How am I going to tell everyone at home?" She said she'd call our auntie Mary Effie Snowshoe and ask her to inform our family members of my results.

 They sent me home, but I was soon sent back to Yellowknife, where they did more tests. While they were doing tests on me, I woke up and they couldn't put me back to sleep. I saw three white things on the screen smaller than a golf ball, and they told me that it was the cancer. They sent me for surgery, but they never gave me an escort to Yellowknife. Yet I noticed the other thirty people sitting in the waiting room had an escort with them. I sat there silently crying because I felt so alone. After this appointment I travelled back home to Fort McPherson. Then soon afterwards I had to travel back to Yellowknife, again on my own with no escort. When I saw the doctor, he asked me where my escort was. "I was told I didn't need one," I said, but he soon got me one anyway — my sister Kathy was able to come with me to my surgery.

The surgery was only supposed to take two or three hours, but it ended up taking ten hours. This was stressful for my family as no one told them anything about why surgery took longer than expected. After that, I had to stay in Yellowknife for two weeks to recover. When we were preparing to leave Yellowknife, I went to get my staples removed. During this appointment, my doctor came to give me my results. She said the surgery was a success and that I didn't need any further treatment except to heal from the surgery. I wasn't even able to sew for the first little while after my surgery. I couldn't do anything except sit. I fell into a depression because of that, and that's when I started going for my little walks outside.

I told my dad that I was okay, and he said, "Mahsi." Then I went home, and my friend Ellen Wilson kept sending for me because she only had a few months to live. When I finally visited her, I just started crying. I told her it was really hard for me to visit her because I was cancer free, and I felt guilty. She said, "That's okay, I lived my life, I taught my girls everything, and I think I was a good mother, so I'm happy." Those were her last words to me. From then on up until today I share my stories with other people and mostly with people who have been diagnosed with cancer.

Many people with cancer come to me and ask me questions. I let them know that even if they are in Edmonton, or Yellowknife on medical, any time they need to talk, I'm here and they can phone me. I'm really happy to share my story with other people and their families who are going through a cancer diagnosis because it's very hard when you are diagnosed with cancer and have no support. Having more support will strengthen you through your journey. I always think of Mary Teya, who told me to "think positive and beat it — don't let it beat you," and that's what I did. I could really feel that people were praying for me when I was in Yellowknife, and I was thankful for that. In return, I try to help people as much as I can. Even though I am a single mother I still share traditional food with others.

I needed someone beside me when I found out I had cancer. I told the doctor afterwards they need to make sure that people have support beside them when they are giving results. He agreed with me, but I don't know if anything has changed. Since I gave that feedback, I know of another person who was told the news that they had cancer while they were all alone. In my journey, I had no professional support other than my family and friends. Today, I still go down South for check-ups, and they still tell me I don't need an escort.

The worst part of finding out I had cancer was not knowing how far along the cancer was and if they were going to be able to get it out. My mom really talked to me; she told me to pray and that God would get me through it. My kids were sad when I was leaving for tests and surgery, but I told them to pray. When I got home after surgery, I walked into my house and my whole family was there. They had a big meal cooked for me, people came to visit, and they brought traditional food. It was like that every day for the first little while when I returned home. Every day I tried walking outside, slowly taking extra steps until I finally made it to the graveyard. I did that every day. I got many phone calls and people prayed with me. When I was strong enough and able to get around, I went on the radio station and thanked people for praying for me and doing good things for me. In return, I try to help people as much as I can.

When I asked the doctor what caused the cancer, he told me that it was processed food, fat from store-bought meat, and not eating my traditional food from the land. There is a lot of pollution on our land. People pick berries on the side of the road, but trucks fly by and chemicals fall on the berries. Mouldy homes can cause cancer too. They know that smoking causes cancer, but smoking is one of the hardest things to quit.

Cancer has made me a better person. I am closer to my family members, siblings, and children. I enjoy life more, especially with my grandchildren. Starting a support group with cancer patients, survivors, and family members is a good way to help. It's a place where we can share our experiences. I really want to start up a support group and share more information on cancer in our community because we don't see any information about cancer here. If I didn't experience cancer myself, I really wouldn't know how to support others affected by cancer.

If someone were to approach me today and tell me they or a loved one was diagnosed with cancer, I would stop and listen to this person. I would invite them to share whatever they need to. I would ask this person if they would like me to continue being there as a support person for them or if I could help to find someone else to support them. Having people around you that you trust is so important.

Agnes Pascal

FORT MCPHERSON

Giving up was not an option for me. It still isn't.

I am from Tetlit Zheh (Fort McPherson), and I was custom adopted by my jijuu (grandmother) Laura and jijii (grandfather) Ronnie Pascal. At the time, they were already elderly, and they had lots of help with my upbringing from all my aunties and uncles, including my mom, Martha Moses. I'm a single parent of two young adults, Ronnie and Laura Pascal, and I have another beautiful daughter, Seanna Heather. I have close connections with my many McPhoo cousins, who are very much like siblings to me. From each of these people, I carry some special teaching from their presence in my life. I've seen a tradition within my family and community, where one chosen grandchild is blessed to be raised by their grandparents. This custom is still practised today, and I'm honoured to have been this grandchild for our Pascal family.

When my children were younger, I decided I wanted to further my education. This meant my family and I would need to move to the Yukon from our home in the Northwest Territories. That was a big change for us. I enrolled in the bachelor of social work program at Yukon College. At the very beginning of the first year of my studies was when my cancer journey began. When I look back now, it all seems so unreal, still. I went to the doctor following up

Agnes, Ronnie, and Laura Pascal with their dogs, Jack and Buddy Pascal. Photo by Tony Devlin.

on a different concern. I had mentioned to my friend that I had felt a lump on my breast, and that friend told me to tell my doctor about it. I would have just shrugged it off, as I knew there could be many reasons for a woman to have a lump on her breast.

At the appointment, my doctor did a quick breast examination and ordered a mammogram screening. Prior to this, I worked in many health offices booking medical appointments for patients. So, I was aware of the risk groups for various cancers, and I wasn't in any of these categories. I felt reassured the doctor was checking this concern. Only a few days after the mammogram, I was called back from the Whitehorse General Hospital Diagnostics Department to book a breast ultrasound appointment. I began to feel concerned — what if it could be cancer? After the ultrasound was complete, I was told a biopsy was needed. I began asking questions at this point: Why are all these follow-up appointments happening with no explanation? During that time, numerous different thoughts and questions were going through my mind. I began praying for all that I needed to carry me through this situation. My doctor came to me afterwards and said, "Don't worry until I tell you it's time to worry." My doctor also told me that the results from the biopsy would take a week or two to come back.

Waiting for my biopsy results was difficult for me. I was very emotional. I went through lots of negative feelings. I wondered, if I have cancer, am I going to die? Who will care for my children, or who would I be able to trust to love my children as I do? I'm a single parent and my children are my biggest concern. During this whole time, I prayed so hard. This gave me peace and by the time I went to my appointment for my results I felt confident that everything was fine. My doctor was running late and I waited in the exam room. I felt better knowing he was late because I thought if he had bad news to give me, he wouldn't have me waiting. When he finally walked in, he appeared in a cheerful mood, humming a tune away. Then he looked at me, and said, "Yup, it's cancer," while slapping my medical chart on the table down in front of me. At that moment, I felt all my energy drain from my body as I just sat there and stared at him. They say that when you hear news like that, your whole life flashes before your eyes. It's true! Then the thought hit me: I'm going to die! I thought of my children and my family, who had no idea that all of this was taking place. At that time, my children were in Inuvik with my parents Martha and Winston Moses.

My doctor began explaining my diagnosis to me. I swear, all I saw was him sitting there with his mouth moving: I heard a word here and there but that was it. Then he began drawing diagrams of lumps that were cancerous. He showed me a diagram of the options I had for surgery. He explained chemotherapy and radiation therapy to me. He told me I would be required to follow through on the surgery of my choice: either a lumpectomy or a mastectomy on my right side. He said that I would require both chemotherapy and radiation after I was healed from surgery. All I did was cry as I listened as best as I could. I felt numb. I was all alone in Whitehorse at that time.

I called a few people close to me and told them the news. I told my auntie Mary Effie Snowshoe, who I always turn to in everything good and bad. When we spoke, I told her that I didn't want people knowing right away. She told me she had to tell others so that they could pray for me. I couldn't argue with that! I was given space as needed from my entire family. I have a close relationship with my Pascal family; they know me very well and they knew exactly what I needed at that time. It was a time when I was coming to terms with a cancer diagnosis, and no cancer patient likes to be questioned regularly. We do this enough with our steady rotation of new physicians and locums in the North, where every time you get a new doctor, they ask questions and more questions. I found it frustrating that most doctors didn't review my file before a medical appointment, as though I was seeing them to treat the common cold, not cancer.

My surgery was scheduled in Whitehorse shortly after my diagnosis. The surgery went well, and I was told I had Yukon's dream team of medical and surgical professionals with me that day! But after surgery, I fell apart many times. Depression was very sneaky and snuck in on me a few times during recovery from surgery. I found myself abusing alcohol even after years of abstinence. By this time Christmas was fast approaching and I arrived back to Inuvik just in time for the holidays.

In early January I went to the Cross Cancer Institute in Edmonton for my first appointment. Little did I know that the Cross Cancer would become one of my favourite places while undergoing cancer treatment. When you enter the Cross Cancer, you are introduced to many individuals who have faced or are battling cancer. They offer you support. You realize we all have the same goal, which is to beat cancer. If a family member was to ask you, "How are you doing?" you would say, "I'm fine," so that this person doesn't worry about you. If someone else who has experienced cancer and knows what it is really like asks how you are doing, you would be much more honest in answering their question. These are the kind of people and the kind of support and comfort I found at the Cross Cancer Institute. This is also where I met with my oncologist, and where he explained my treatment plan to me. He mentioned that concerns with my lymph nodes would cause me to proceed with treatment quicker than we all anticipated.

Ruth Wright was my escort at this time. Thank goodness I had her by my side as I found myself feeling very emotional during this visit. Ruth was able to ask the doctor good questions on my behalf before proceeding further with treatment. I cried when he confirmed that I would be losing my hair. My treatment plan included six rounds of chemotherapy, then a six-week break, followed by five to six weeks of radiation treatment. During the first visit to the Cross Cancer, I received my first round of chemo; the remaining five would be administered in Yellowknife.

Just the sound of the word chemotherapy is scary, or at least, it scared me. I didn't know what to expect. I was afraid of negative side effects that I heard about. My worries calmed on the day of my first chemo. I was hooked up to an IV that administered the chemo, a process which took about an hour or two. That part was no problem. Slowly but surely the side effects would come by evening the same day. I had no appetite, so I drank meal replacement drinks and traditional broth. Other side effects of chemo like fatigue and nausea decreased as the days passed leading up to the next scheduled round of treatment. I don't know what I dreaded more: the chemotherapy or having to travel again.

I can recall a period after my surgery, and when I was beginning chemotherapy, where I began experiencing pain in different areas of my body. I was prescribed pain medication, adding to my already large amount of prescribed medication. Shortly after, I noticed I was feeling drained, fatigue, and weak. This worried me, so I followed up with a medical appointment to discuss that feeling because I couldn't cope with it. I was worried as a single mom whose children were fully dependent on her between treatment medical trips. I couldn't be so tired all the time. I needed to be there for them.

The doctor I saw asked why I was put on this medication. I replied, "For pain." He explained that the pills were antidepressants, something I had always stayed away from. I had a large bag of medication. I didn't know what half of them were for, and some carried side effects that were hard on me and my system. I suffered with severe dry skin. My friend who suffered with another disease told me about how medical cannabis helped him. I had experience smoking weed recreationally now and then, and I chose to use medical cannabis for the remainder of my treatment. I'm not influencing anyone to do the same, but I found it helpful.

After my diagnosis, life continued. There were many hardships to overcome, not just cancer. I couldn't commit to any jobs. I had to go on income support and disability insurance. It hurt my pride to do this as I had always worked and taken care of my children, but as the side effects of chemotherapy were setting in, I couldn't work anymore. The side effects were rough at times, but not all the time. Just when I would feel better for a day or two, I would be off for my next round.

I remember when my fourth one was coming up and I was dreading it. I made up my mind that I didn't want to do chemo anymore. I was feeling better. I felt okay about my decision to stop. I knew I would have to explain my decision to my aunts and uncles, and they'd understand, but the thought of the look in their eyes if I told them I was giving up on chemo was not worth it. They didn't raise me to come this far only to stop now. That thought alone gave me the push I needed to continue with treatment and finish all six rounds. I remembered who Agnes Pascal is: I'm a strong person who will get through cancer. Knowing that also gave me the strength and encouragement I needed not to give up.

Each time I had to travel for medical to Edmonton or Yellowknife, I was fortunate to have an escort. I can't stress enough the importance of having an escort during those visits. I chose escorts who knew me well because you need someone who knows you well enough to understand what you're going through and not take your bad mood personally. You need someone who can speak for you and ask good medical questions to your doctors. Someone you feel comfortable with in your space to care for you in between visits to your doctor. Heather was my main escort for medical travel. I had other escorts too, whose patience I tested to their limits with my stubbornness. But with Heather, we always had memorable adventures on these trips for treatment. She always had good questions for the cancer care team.

My brother, Alfred Moses, was MLA for the riding of Inuvik Boot Lake during this time. He always took time from his busy schedule to ensure Heather and I were okay. He checked in with us every time we went to Edmonton. Most times he would send us out for a nice supper in the city. That is how Alfred cared for his family and community. Alfred was a go-getter at whatever he challenged and succeeded at. He was so excited that *Book of Hope* was in the works and suggested that it be published in all our languages of the Northwest Territories. His dream was to travel and explore new adventures; he loved travelling. He has since passed.

My parents cared for my children when I was away. My son was younger then, and one day I noticed he was going somewhere each evening. I asked my mom and she said, "He's going to church." I felt so happy. My jijuu always prayed with us and taught us the importance of having faith and to pray. When I found out he was going to church, I felt sad that he was going alone. One morning, I decided to go with him. Then more family members started attending church too! This was a blessing given to us all from my son. During this time, my own faith was growing. I prayed to God and said, "I really don't understand why this is happening to me, but you do, and I'm trusting you." I told him I wanted to live a life where I can see my children grow up and have families of their own, and that I wanted to have lots of grandchildren to spoil with love too.

On March 24 I was told that treatment was a success. I cried and felt as if heavy weights were lifted off my shoulders. I was in a state of complete joy. You don't remember all the dark stages of your treatment in that moment. I thanked God for his healing, I know it was Him. From then on, I was told I would only have to continue with follow-up visits to the doctor. Life was great!

But each time I would travel for a follow-up appointment, I could feel fear setting within me. I begin to think, "What if they tell me it's back?" One November visit, my fear became reality. I was told that the cancer was back and that when cancer returns, it can be aggressive and spread quickly. Then they told me that I'd have to begin the whole chemo and radiation process over again but at a faster pace. Of course,

I cried. I thought about how happy my children were when I told them that my cancer was gone and to have to tell them that it was back was heartbreaking. I knew I had to depend on my faith. I thought of the Book of Isaiah, and the command to not fear, for God is with me: He will strengthen and help me. I knew even in the darkest times I am not forsaken. I began praying and believed I would be healed again. I told my doctor, "Just watch, you'll see, I'll beat it again by believing."

There was an intense treatment plan put in place for me. I did not tell anyone because it was during the Christmas holiday season, and I didn't want to darken anyone's spirits. We were celebrating the first Christmas of a few babies within our Pascal family that year, too. After the holidays I met with my surgeon in Inuvik to discuss treatment plans. I mentioned that I knew I was there to discuss my treatment plan. She sat with a puzzled look on her face. She said that she was checking and rechecking all my results to be certain. Then she said, "Your cancer is gone, just gone, with no explanation." I said, "I told you it's the power of prayer for healing." She said, "Whatever it is, I hope you share this as we have no explanation as to why it's gone. Praise God!" she said excitedly. That's when I began telling others about what happened. Family members were upset that I never told them right away that I had cancer again.

Since I was diagnosed, my family is more aware of cancer. Unfortunately, I'm not the only family member who fought to battle cancer in our family. Sadly, experience with cancer in our family started with my jijii Ronnie shortly after I was born. He passed away years later from his illness. Later down the road we lost my auntie Agnes, who my jijii Ronnie named me after. We lost my uncle James to colon cancer. He and my auntie Edith's children now have to be screened for cancer every five years. Then it was my uncle Michael Pascal Sr., who was a father to me all my life. It was hard saying goodbye to him and maddening to see what this ugly sickness can do. I am grateful that I had the opportunity to tell him how thankful I am for him and that I loved him. Cancer does give you the opportunity to have closure. I know he was proud of me, and he encouraged me in all I did. There are quite a few survivors of cancer in our family today, and some still battling this disease

I'm the type of person who knows there's light at the end of the tunnel and good always arises out of bad. Cancer has changed my life for the better. I don't stress over little things anymore. I take each day as a blessing and as an opportunity to be a better person and mother. I met loads of beautiful people along the way who I would have never known if it hadn't been for cancer. When I was struggling alone at times during my journey, I realized the importance of having support. Along with family members, caregivers need a tremendous amount of support to cope. I attended a one-time cancer support group held in Inuvik and saw and felt the difference that connecting with other cancer patients on a personal level can make. I then began our own cancer support group here in Inuvik in 2018. We meet monthly to do all sorts of activities, but mostly sharing circles. Ruth Wright, my medical travel advocate, and Mary Roland both help to run our group. I want to continue to encourage and support others who need that extra friend who cares. I'm challenging myself by working towards a Northern Indigenous Counselling Diploma to gain strong tools to be a better supporter and helper of our people.

I was fortunate, along with group members Ruth Wright and Mary Roland, to attend the World Indigenous Cancer Conference in Calgary in 2019 through our funders Hotıì ts'eeda.[1] At this conference Daryl Fox shared about his brother, Terry Fox, on such a personal level that tears came to the eyes of many of us in the audience. He shared that his brother did not once feel sorry for himself but instead used what he was going through to educate us all about cancer. He began one of Canada's largest foundations that all of us touched by cancer can feel grateful for today. Because of research, many of us can beat cancer today. Mr. Fox shared that if Terry were to be diagnosed today with the same cancer, he would have survived without losing any limbs. We should all give to these foundations and spread awareness that a cancer diagnosis is not a death sentence: you have hope of survival. God Bless and mahsi.

Note

1   Hotıì ts'eeda is the Canadian Institutes of Health Research–funded Strategy for Patient Oriented Research support unit for the Northwest Territories. Since it was established in 2018, it has funded and supported many community-based health initiatives across the NWT.

Mary Effie Snowshoe

FORT MCPHERSON

I am from Fort McPherson, and my husband is the late Charlie Snowshoe, a well-respected Elder of Fort McPherson. My parents are the late Ronnie and Laura Pascal. All our children are on their own now, with their own families.

I never attended residential school. The main reason I didn't attend was that my parents lost children who attended residential school. They died. This story was told to me over and over: my parents sent two children to residential school in Hay River and they never returned home.[1] My dad recalls my sister Louisa was 5 or 6 years of age, and my brother John was age 3 or 4 when they left home to go to residential school. At first, they told him they were only taking the little girl. My dad disagreed and didn't want to let her leave. Those days no one really understood law and people were scared of RCMP. Also, our people never spoke the English language. But these people had translators with them. My dad repeatedly shook his head and disagreed with them taking his daughter, my sister Louisa. He was told that if he didn't send his children to residential school he could go to jail. Going to jail scared him, and he didn't know what jail was. Finally, he gave in to them and told them if you're going to take my daughter, you take my son too. Because I don't want her to be alone.

Photo by Arlyn Charlie.

Seeing them leaving home really hurt my mom and dad. My dad recalls memories of seeing the boat leaving, and his son John looked back at my parents standing on the shore. John started crying, then my parents began to cry too as the boat left and they could no longer see the boat or hear John crying. My dad always told this story and says when he heard his son cry from the boat, it was the last cry he ever heard from him, because he never returned home. All I heard was that they both passed away around the age they had left.

When my dad told this story in the late 1950s, he said to me, "I'll never forget that my two kids never came back. I signed the paper when they told me I could go to jail." But he didn't sign his name, he signed with an X. My mother signed her name as well by printing an X. This was one reason my dad never let me attend residential school. My brother and sister were both buried at Hay River with no option of remains being sent back home to Fort McPherson. My dad purchased headstones for both of my siblings, and they were placed on their graves at the old grave site in Hay River.

I had another sister who was older than me, she was named Louisa too! I was around the age of 5 or 6 at this time. I remember my dad telling me that my sister Louisa was leaving and would be away for long time. I asked him where she was going. "She'll be going to All Saints school in Aklavik," he answered. I started crying when he told me. I asked If I could go with her too. He told me, "No, I'm not sending you." My dad said that he lost too many children, but he's sending Louisa this time. My sister Louisa went to Aklavik in September. Her remains were returned to my dad the following January. I was 6 years old when she died. I'll be 86 this year, yet today I still don't know the cause of my sister's death. This was the only time that I've ever heard my dad really cry, during the 1950s when he lost his children to attend residential school. I still have questions about my older sister's death in Aklavik, and we've never received any type of report back of how she died. I was very lucky that my dad chose not to send me to school during these times.

By this time, I was six and a half years of age. I only spoke my language; I didn't know or understand one word of English. Not even simple words such as thank you, yes, or no. I was told I was sick — I had this disease I've never heard of before called TB or tuberculosis. My sister Agnes was given same diagnosis at this time too. They sent us to

Aklavik All Saints Hospital. When I hear stories of Aklavik Residential School, All Saints Hospital treated children the same way. I went through hard times there. I couldn't speak English. We went in this big building that I'd never seen before. I started eating food I'd never eaten before. I cried and cried and I don't know how many times I got slapped by nurses for crying. I'll always remember how they used to bring me a cup of black broth to drink and tell me to drink it even though it didn't taste good. It helped if you drank water afterwards to help it go down. I didn't know what this liquid was. I asked my sister Agnes in our language, "What are they giving me?" She said that it was medicine for TB. When I knew the nurse was coming with medication, I would shake my head to indicate I don't want this medication. Often my hair would be grabbed and my head pulled back so they could pour the liquid down my throat. After being forced to take the medication, I would cry. When I cried, I would get slapped by one of these workers. Years later, my sister Agnes documented and recorded these stories of our experiences of Aklavik Residential School and All Saints Hospital. She has since passed. There were many times she would tell me, "Don't cry or they're going to slap you again." This was my daily experience at this hospital.

My name is Mary and Gwich'in say "mare-eee." While in Aklavik Hospital, I was never called Mary or Mare-eee by the head nurse. She called me "Indian kid." I don't understand what she meant by Indian kid. Even when speaking to other nurses about me, she would point to me and say, Indian kid. I heard this so many times as a young child. I believed that my name was Indian kid and I felt kind of proud of that word, which I didn't understand. Yet, I was confused because I thought my name was Mary. I finally went home after two and half years in All Saints Hospital when I was 9 years old. Before returning home, I finally learned what Indian kid meant after being called this name for all these years, from the All Saints Hospital's head nurse. Today we don't use the word Indian; we use Gwich'in People, Aboriginal People, Indigenous People.

I knew what she meant. I thought to myself, "This Indian kid is going to show you white people who's an Indian kid." Do you know what I got out of that? I got the power to show them that this Indian kid is going to be a very smart woman. I pushed myself to gain knowledge from my people, Elders, and my parents. I got valuable teachings from them. They taught me how to survive off the land. How important our land and culture are to us. I have all these teachings from all these Elders and my parents that I now share with those who want to learn these skills. All my Elders who taught me should be given the credit for sharing their knowledge and passing this on to me. I share this knowledge with others; I don't keep it. All these teaching helped me to be who I am today: a smart Indian kid.

Growing up, I never heard of cancer. The worst sickness that lots of people were dying from at that time was TB. I got married in 1960 at age 22. I was in my early 30s when I heard they were going to begin treating our drinking water. I was approached by one of my Southern friends who told me, "Mary, I don't like that they are going to begin treating your water." He said, "Down the line this may cause cancer." That was when I heard of cancer. I asked him, "What is cancer?" He said, "It's a very bad sickness. It kills people." Since then, I avoid drinking tap water. Until two years ago I only drank melted snow and water from the mountains. That's all. The past two years I haven't made it out there to get my water, so I had to drink the tap water that is given to us. Gradually, I did hear of people being sick with cancer. It was then that I recalled my conversation with my Southern friend who warned me about drinking treated water.

I keep track of people I know with cancer. Cancer does kill. I lost my dad Ronnie, my brother Michael, and my sister Agnes to cancer. Nowadays there is a good chance to beat cancer if you get checked right away. In the past, long ago you never heard of cancer, just TB, and people lived long lives, some into their late 90s or even over 100 years old. Now we don't see people live this long. But I know that if people see their nurse or doctor right away, they have a better chance to survive. We don't understand cancer, so when we see someone ready to pass away from cancer, yes, we're going to get scared.

This is the second time now I have gotten a cancer diagnosis. My first time hearing that I had cancer, I thought, "I'm going to be gone." I got scared. I think I might have cried once. I believe in God so much. I prayed. I knew people were praying for me. People spoke of traditional medicine to me and that's what I did. I used traditional medicine and survived. That was twenty or thirty years ago. I was told that cancer can come back in seven years' time but I made it to now. Now they told me I have cancer again. It's the same experience as last time; I got scared and cried. But through my faith, I believe things will work out. I'm currently using traditional medicine until I go to Edmonton Cross Cancer and meet my oncologist and learn more from there.

When someone comes to me to let me know they have cancer, and they're feeling bad, I know how bad they're feeling from my own experience. First thing I'll share with this person is, leave it into God's hands and let God take care of it; you're going to be okay. Pray, find strength in God, and you're going to be okay.

I would also recommend traditional medicine. It's important to know what stage cancer is in before using traditional medicine. Traditional medicine works good for early stages of cancer. We get prescribed medication from our doctors and use that together with traditional medicine. But there are times when prescribed and traditional medicines don't work together. As well make sure the person making traditional medicine is aware of any environmental allergies. Let's say if you have seasonal allergies to birch but then you go to the bush during the time you're allergic to birch to pick, clean, and prepare spruce gum for yourself and drink it. You will be around a lot of birch and that's not good; you're feeding your sickness and it can cause you to get sicker.

I keep positive thoughts. I have worked with many people of all ages throughout my life helping teach our culture, language, and traditions. Many of them have thanked me; many of them said thank you for being a part of me, thank you for taking me, teaching me. Some share that I've told many stories that have helped others feel good. When I hear these comments, it gives me more power. I tell myself, "I'm not giving up until it's my end."

Note

1   Hay River residential school was also called All Saints, and it was run by the Anglican Mission.

Elizabeth Vittrekwa

FORT MCPHERSON

I'm married to Peter James Vittrekwa, and I have five children and four grandchildren. I'm from Fort McPherson. I'm Tetlit Gwich'in. My parents are Charlie and Mary Effie Snowshoe of Fort McPherson.

In February 2020 when the COVID-19 pandemic hit, I was scheduled for a second mammogram in Yellowknife. I rescheduled that appointment due to the fear of COVID-19, and I made it to Yellowknife the following July. There were concerns, but I said I wasn't going through with the biopsy. I'm okay with it. Then, I remember, I was driving around. My grandson asked me, "Jijuu, what you had to go to Yellowknife for?" Then he asked when am I going out again. That pushed me to do the biopsy.

I was sent to Edmonton for a breast biopsy. I travelled all alone to my biopsy appointment. I was told I would get an escort to accompany me but until the last minute before travelling, I was fighting for an escort. When I was going to meet with my doctor to discuss my diagnosis, we had to fight for my husband to accompany me as my escort. After the biopsy procedure, I was told that the results would take five to ten days. I returned back North. While I was in isolation by myself, the doctor confirmed breast cancer. At this time, I was in mandatory isolation in Inuvik for two weeks.

Elizabeth and Peter James Vittrewka.

After my isolation period was over, Peter James and I travelled to Edmonton to follow up with my doctor. My doctor explained the breast cancer to us. He said there were two lumps. One lump was stage 2 cancer. The other was cancerous, but not as invasive as the first lump. But this second lump would eventually become invasive. There was a third lump too, but they were not concerned about it. They began the process immediately to remove both lumps.

When I told people other than my family members, someone told me to "be positive." Then someone told me that I'm a strong person, but I didn't feel like I was. My cousin Andrew told me, "Liz, you've got to have faith." That was what carried me through was faith. I didn't feel strong and I didn't have positive thoughts. The different emotions I was experiencing were a challenge, but it was faith that carried me through. Many times I fell apart. It was my dad who said, "My girl, if you're OK, we will be OK." I had to tell family members that I needed their strength to help me. I told them that if we all stay strong together, we will all build on our strengths together.

There was also my cousin Agnes Pascal and my friend Annalee from Aklavik; they walked me through what to expect. So, with both of them by my side, saying, "Okay, this is what's going to happen with a biopsy," and so forth, and walking me through all those steps of what to expect. Other than them there was nobody. After my surgery in Edmonton, I was then contacted by the Northwest Territories cancer navigators.[1] An Alberta nurse followed up with me and supplied resources. But when you just came out of surgery, you don't feel like looking at resource material. It would have been more helpful to have all these resources ahead of time! I was fortunate to have my two supports, but I'm sure there are people out there who don't have others to turn to. It was only after everything was over that the cancer navigation team called me.

My surgery was scheduled during the pandemic. This meant that the regular flight schedules had changed. We left Fort McPherson for Inuvik, which is a two-hour drive. Then catch our flight to Edmonton. If we're lucky, after arriving in Edmonton, they accommodate us at Larga Home with a cold supper waiting for us. We were fortunate that we were sent money to buy supper that evening. That's a long day, and you're full of anxiety. Your appointment is early the next morning. You suffer from jet lag and can't sleep dealing with all these anxieties. By early dawn, I was then preparing for another full day, including my surgery. Because of the pandemic, Peter James wasn't able to come to the hospital with me. So, Peter James and I had to say our goodbyes at Larga Home that morning. Then I was dropped off for my surgery by a Larga Home bus driver, who couldn't even take me into the hospital.

I was told my surgery would be an hour and a half, followed by two hours in the recovery room. Nobody told me anything besides that. Before this my mom had told me "as soon as you wake up, start moving your toes and hands until you can walk." So, I did that. I was given oxygen during this time after my surgery. I never left the hospital until five that evening. I wasn't told why I was there that long. After the nurse saw that I could walk, and I was doing okay, I was discharged. Peter James was there to pick me up with the Larga Home bus driver. COVID rules meant that the nurse walked me to the door where my husband waited for me. We were supposed to return back to Inuvik the following day, but my husband changed our flights and we paid for another hotel room for a few days, which was good because I ended up in the emergency room in Edmonton in the early hours.

When we got back, we went right into isolation for two weeks. The first time I went to Edmonton for my biopsy, I went right into fourteen-day isolation when I got back. One day of freedom from isolation. Then I travelled back South, then went back into isolation. Three times in a row we did that. It was hard on me. It was truly hard on me. I thank God for family and friends in Inuvik. My friends and family cooked traditional foods and brought it to me at the Mackenzie Hotel, where we were in isolation. This was so important because there were no traditional food or meals offered by the Mackenzie Hotel to us First Nations people in isolation who are used to these foods in our daily diet. Then, I was placed at Capital Suites because I couldn't climb the stairs at the Mackenzie Hotel. But we were told that our daily meals would be our responsibility. So, thank God for our family and friends who cooked for us and sent us food. After this my isolation plan was approved so I could stay at my cabin outside Fort McPherson, and we did move to our cabin.

During the pandemic, it was a real struggle to fight with medical travel. It is unbelievable. It adds to the stress you're already experiencing with cancer having to fight for an escort. It's the worst thing being alone and being told that you have cancer. That is the worst thing.

I'm so used to doing things on my own and being independent, but after my surgery, Peter James had to help me lots. I cried and he asked, "What's wrong?" I told him that I didn't like this, "I don't like my surgery. I don't like losing my independence. I want everything back!" We talked about it. Then I spoke to one of my community Elders, who talked and prayed with me. I called Agnes to talk. I then called another friend who experienced this type of cancer. She shared with me that, because of my surgery, I was losing something. She mentioned that my body has to grieve for that! That was part of you for all your life she said. She walked me through the steps. So, in times like that I try to utilize all my supports. With them, we got through a lot of emotional, physical, and mental challenges.

I wasn't told that I had to watch for the cold afterwards. I was reading a book and questioned one of the cancer navigators about it. She then went through this book with me and answered my questions. Like about wound cuts, and my blood pressure, not taking tests on the side of your cancer. Having to wash your hands regularly during the pandemic caused my hands to become very dry and cracked. I have to be careful with that. There are lots of areas that I have to be careful about.

Truth be told, I get sick of reading about cancer. I tell myself when I wake up in the mornings that "I'm not sick." I don't want cancer to consume my life. People stop me on the street and say, "Liz, how are you doing?" When asked questions, I find that I end up talking in depth about cancer. I let them know that I try not to speak of it lots because of my faith. I believe that I'm healed. Especially as a woman, cancer alters your life to accommodate this sickness. With the pills I take, I go through all these different emotions. The pills are there to fight to ensure that no cancer cells grow within my body. But then I deal with hot flashes and fatigue as side effects. It's hard. I really watch the way I think, but it's hard. I thank God for Peter James 'cause he hears all this. He talks me through it or lets me vent. Then afterwards he asks how I'm feeling and if I'm going to be okay. Just hearing those words and knowing someone is there with you helps.

I have a big family. I know people who had breast cancer within the community. Members of our community would share their experiences with cancer with my mom, Mary Effie Snowshoe. She then relayed all these stories to me. When I was going to Edmonton in September to meet with my doctor for the first time, I have six siblings who gave us money. They told us to use the money however we wanted. They gave me a little pep talk before I left for Edmonton. There again, I cried! I felt my independence was being taken because I had to rely on other people financially. The second time I travelled, they made sure I was okay financially too.

One thing about our community too, was they prayed for me. People from the church prayed for me. People were phoning and praying with me. My family, community members, and Elders would come up to me and give me a hug. Then in November, we had a family dinner. I went around the community delivering plates of food to Elders. One of the Elders told me, "Oh my God, I didn't think I'd see you walking in my house." I told her that I was okay. Even at the airport, lots of people were coming up to me and giving me a hug and telling me that I'll be okay. I think I'm lucky. I truly am, because I have all these people here praying for me. I'm fortunate!

My children, who are all grown, helped me too. With my family I hid nothing. I was honest with them. I explained my surgery and what was going to happen. Right down to my grandson and my granddaughters, I explained everything. After all this I tell them to watch their bodies and make sure they check themselves monthly. It can happen to anyone. But because it happened to me, we all have to be extra careful. Even my sisters and my mom I tell the same thing to. My mom had colon cancer. They are aware they should watch for all types. Anyone who asks me questions regarding breast cancer, if I have the answer, I will share with them. It's really hard because at times I feel really self-conscious. A nurse told me that when she sees someone like me, it reminds her of her grandmother and she thinks of strength. She said, "Don't be self-conscious Liz, and think of your strength. What you went through wasn't easy," and it wasn't. So, I do have to remind myself and say that it's okay. My sister Shirley told me about Terry Fox. She said that before he began his run, the percentage of people dying from cancer was high. Today the percentage of cancer deaths is lower. Hearing this type of encouragement gave me strength. Thank God for people who send me messages to not be hard on myself. Like, "You are going to feel fatigue. Just take it as it comes." So that's what I do daily.

During the pandemic, you couldn't give hugs. But with anybody experiencing this, just give them a hug and show that you care and remind them to have faith. I don't want to tell them to be strong or be positive. Because right at that moment your world is just turning, turning upside down. I know for myself, I went on the internet and because of my faith I would pick healing verses. Even gospel songs, I wouldn't listen to sad gospel songs. I looked for uplifting gospel songs. That's what I listened to. I went through this; there's lots of people gone through this. The odds are in our favour. Even now, I am telling others to watch for anything concerning and get it checked. Be persistent. Make sure you have a medical escort with you, don't do it alone. I'll be here to help in any way. Like what Agnes and Annalee did for me, by going step by step with me, by saying this is how it's going to be, this might happen, and the resources are here.

My cancer was unique. The doctor initially told me that I'll be on pills and have to do radiation therapy. Afterwards in October, they called and told me that the cancer never spread. But I would still have to take pills and chemotherapy. I couldn't see myself doing this. I cried with my siblings and asked them to pray that I don't have to do chemotherapy. I had long discussions with Cross Cancer Institute to avoid chemo. They got my approval to send my tumours down to California for further testing. They called and said the cancer percentage was low so doing chemotherapy wouldn't have made much difference. I only take pills now. That's where I say, "All the glory is given to God," because that's what we prayed for. I didn't have to do chemotherapy. I don't like talking about it, 'cause I know there's someone right now receiving chemo.

There are people out there with no support. Like right now there's no cancer support in our community, nothing like the Inuvik Cancer Support Group. I spoke to an Elder and shared how I felt. He said, "That's the way it is." I think support groups are needed in every community, especially when you are experiencing hard days. Even though we look strong on the outside, on the inside we're fighting our own battles. During this pandemic I lost my cousin from pancreatic cancer in June. I didn't have a chance to grieve for her. Then in December my uncle John Eds was sent to Inuvik. He was diagnosed with lung cancer and passed away. It was such a trial to go through all this. I wonder, could all this be avoided if their cancer had been detected sooner? Or if we had more advanced medical equipment? We should be entitled to have the good equipment within the Northwest Territories to detect cancer sooner.

Note

1   The Cancer Navigator Program helps cancer patients to navigate the health care system. It is made up of a team of two nurses and a social worker. The program is provided by the NWT Health and Social Services Authority.

Ernest Vittrekwa

FORT MCPHERSON

I was born in Aklavik seventy-seven years ago. Back in the fifties I moved to Fort McPherson. All my life, I lived on the land. I went through all kinds of sickness. Them days there were no hospitals, unlike now. We used to stay on the land when sick and relied on what we had, like spruce gum juice and other traditional medicine. We ate food off the land. It was a good life.

Both my parents were infected with tuberculosis while I was attending residential school in Aklavik. I was sort of considered an orphan during that time. I was placed here and there. My dad tried to provide food by hunting for me and my three sisters. So, we were all over the place here and there. I was raised this way until I turned fourteen when I began working for myself. I learned to be independent, and I'm still like this today. I live day by day.

I worked hard and never thought of cancer. I remember one year that I walked on snowshoes towards Dawson, Yukon Territory, through five feet of snow.[1] I never saw the others behind me; they were on ski-doo all day. I kept ahead of them. Back then I smoked lots too. Another guy walked ahead of us in five feet of snow, and he smoked too. He left a cigarette butt trail for us over the mountains through deep snow.

Photo by Tony Devlin.

One year we went to Old Crow, Yukon, on our annual community trip by ski-doo. I couldn't even crank my ski-doo. I still can't crank it; I had no energy. We got to Curtain Mountain and camped there. When I got up that morning, I went to start my ski-doo. It wouldn't start. It was frozen. But I never got excited. Me and Alice just stayed at the cabin, made tea, and sat around. We were safe there anyways. Alice was sewing inside the cabin. I prayed and went to try to start the ski-doo again. It was cold out. It was just like when I went into NorthMart and got a new ski-doo.[2] I put the key in and started it, nothing wrong with it! God helped me, it's the truth. 'Cause, I went to heaven. It's hard for me to talk about it, 'cause people don't believe me. I've been there and it's all still in my memory, and that's what keeps me going.

Twelve years ago, all of sudden I started getting tired while I was trapping. The tiredness continued, and then I began getting pains in my stomach. I was getting stomach aches. Even so, I never gave up and I kept trapping, trapping. Then I found I couldn't even sit on my ski-doo. I would stand all day in pain, doing my work. I would tough it out, thinking it was due to getting older in age. I found that I was sleeping more, which I never did before, but I wasn't sick. I went for a check-up and had tests done in Edmonton. My wife Alice was with me through all this.

The doctor said I had cancer. I never got excited. Alice was right there while I was talking to the doctor. I told the doctor — the doctor that Alice and I know now — I told him, "You, as the doctor, will have to do the best you can with me. I'll pray." I can remember telling him this; I wasn't scared or nothing. We were staying at Larga Home, and it was only afterwards that having cancer hit me! Alice was very patient and understanding with me. I went for a long walk alone and said a prayer. I knew it was going to be okay if I kept praying. When I returned to Larga, Alice and I decided who we were going to tell about my diagnosis. Telling my daughter Laura was very hard, and we asked her partner to tell her. Then my sister-in-law Mary Teya, then shared with the rest of the family in Fort McPherson. One day I shared with Alice on a short walk that for some reason I feel James Ross is going to come around. By this time news of my illness was shared all over. Soon after supper that evening, who walked in the door? James Ross. He took us out and we drove around Edmonton for the evening. Both Alice and I felt good to see James. He changed his flight to come see me in Edmonton. This was what we both needed, to see someone from home.

This was a shock because all I went to Edmonton for was to get an x-ray done and go home. Then I was told I would have to stay in Edmonton and complete cancer treatment. So we stayed. We had our children all back home. Alice and I left everything in God's hands, and I accepted everything. I continued with chemotherapy treatment from February to May. Then I went through a major operation, which took a lot out of me, but I toughed it out. I was too weak; I had no strength. I just hung on! Just took it little by little. That's how I made it through and never gave up. Alice knew that I felt like giving up at times. This was shortly after the doctor had told me that I had couple of days to live. I accepted it! My brother-in-law Joe and his wife Glenda were there with us when the doctor told us this news. Alice cried when the doctor said, "There's nothing more we can do," and Joe and Glenda were a big support for us in Edmonton.

Before the operation something happened to me. I had a vision. I saw hell. I saw people, I saw burning, and I heard yelling. All of this was negative stuff. Then I went to heaven. First person I saw there was my mother-in-law, Alice's mother. She passed away many years before Alice and I got married or were even together. Yet, she asked, "How is Alice?" I told her that the whole family is okay. Lots of them that passed on were there. My mother and father were there too, waving at me. There was a big Bible and God was standing there. There was the most beautiful colour blue, some type of bright blue surrounded by beautiful land. Then before my operation I asked my doctor for a minute to say a prayer. Then I gave the anaesthesiologist the go ahead to put me to sleep.

They removed half of my stomach during my operation. The next day after my operation, I awoke at five in the morning. I didn't have any pain. My doctor came to see me and asked if I was in pain. I said, "Nothing." He said, "Really?" "Although I need to go to the washroom," I told him. He helped me. I needed a wheelchair. He showed me a picture on his iPad — it had the colour that I saw in heaven, clear and bright blue. He told me, "At three o'clock this morning, while you were asleep, ten doctors were studying your x-ray. The white spots showed where cancer was in your body yesterday. We were going to send you back to Inuvik with the expectation of two days to live." He then said,

"Something happened at three o'clock this morning, the white and black spots turned to this colour," and pointed out the clear bright blue on the iPad. My doctor then asked me what I experienced during that time. I told him that I was on a journey. He said, "Oh yeah, I know what you mean. No wonder," he said. "It's a miracle." God always answers my prayers, and I asked him to take all the negative stuff away.

I never got excited. I saw my grandchildren too one time; they were heading towards open water. It's dangerous to do that. I tried calling out to them but they never heard me. I had a revolver in my hand. It was clear ice all around them too. I looked at my grandchildren, then I threw the gun on the ice. I even heard the gun hit the ice. Then I looked and saw my grandchildren crawling towards me. God showed me his gifts: my grandchildren.

I was positive, I had determination. This one day there at Larga Home, I got up early one morning. I called Alice to help me to go to the washroom. She asked, "Why?" I told her that I couldn't walk anymore. This affected me from my waist down. This was why I went on the plane by forklift. Alice helped me. I was in a wheelchair, then walker, soon a cane. I purposely left my cane in my truck; it's still in there, I guess. Look at that, twelve years since my chemotherapy, and my feet are still affected by chemo. Although I didn't lose any hair.

I used a wheelchair on my medicals. Like I said, I had to be forklifted on and off the plane when I travelled. Travelling took a lot out of me. I don't know if everyone understands how difficult it is for a cancer patient to be travelling lots and the long flights to and from your appointments and the drive home to Fort McPherson as well. And we are Elders.

When I was ready to travel home to the Northwest Territories. I requested to stop in Yellowknife for few days. I have a daughter in Yellowknife who I can stay with. The trip was too long, and I had to be put on and taken off the plane with a forklift. I remained positive and didn't give up. Once I started healing, I was in lots of pain. I was given pills to help. But today, I only take two pills. One is for high blood pressure and other for prostate, that's it. I experienced a lot during this time, I tell you. One time my brother-in-law, Joe Charlie, was with me. During this time, I felt like giving up. I prayed for strength and made it through. I then went through radiation, which was tough. I made it through that as well. They must have given me strong radiation therapy 'cause I could feel it.

I asked Alice to call my daughter Laura. Midway Lake Music Festival[3] was going on at this time also. I know they kept people updated during my surgery up at Midway Lake Festival. One guy said when hearing the updates at Midway, "He's coming back."

We came back during the springtime when all the carnivals were starting.[4] Alice and I were stuck at home because of my health. I told Alice, "Let's go to Inuvik." She asked, "Who will drive us to Inuvik?" I told her that I would, and we went to Inuvik. At times I felt pulling where I had my surgery. Later that night, we left Inuvik and went to Aklavik, then home to Fort McPherson. Three days in a row, I travelled to Aklavik. All this time, I was praying. That's the way I fought cancer. I went through pain at times, but I never gave up. I kept doing what made me happy. You can't give up! I never did go back to Edmonton.

I had lots of support and that gave me lots of strength, lots. It was twelve years ago, and I'm still here. I still pray. I got help from all over, I tell you! Even one minister that I know from Vancouver had heard I was in Edmonton. He flew to Edmonton to come see me. When I was there a medicine man came to see me too. Right to this day, good things come my way. When I need help, help comes my way. Main thing is determination.

Alice and I were fortunate to travel together to all my appointments. This one time I wanted to go to my camp at Eight Miles, but I had to be brought back to town. I got too weak. Finally, I made it back to Eight Miles. I wanted to set net, but I couldn't! I was still too weak, it was hard. I rested lots on the couch. Slowly, each day I tried to get up. I made progress daily in moving around. I made it down the hill. My grandson helped me into the boat. I slowly made my way to the back of the boat to start the motor. I had just enough strength to start it! That's how I started fishing again too, by crawling around. He always helped me get my legs into the boat. I fought all the way through.

Some people get excited and give up right away. If God is going to take you, he's going to take you! I always pray. I was one of the lucky ones. I was raised up by my grandfather, Andrew Kunnizzie. He was a mechanic. The house I was raised in is still there halfway to Aklavik; my grandfather raised me there since I was five. Later on, I looked after them. My grandparents took me all the time while I was growing up. Today I'm rewarded with his place halfway to Aklavik.

If I found out someone had a cancer diagnosis, I'll ask and invite them in to talk about it. If they choose to come in, I'll sit with them. I'll ask how they're feeling or ask something to get them to start talking. They do have to talk about it. If they cry, I need to encourage them because this is their time. I give them my time. They have been just told they have cancer; it's important that they talk and cry. It's important for them to know I'm there for them. I'll see if I can help in any way. Sometimes we have to accept things that we can't handle, that's what I did. I listened and did all that the doctor ordered me to do. They knew what they were doing. When you don't listen to doctor's orders, then it causes other areas to get out of line too! I've seen this happen to some patients. You just got to accept the things you can't change and have courage to change the things you can.

Don't give up, don't give up! Try to be positive all the time. Giving up is not going to make things better! Be positive with determination.

Notes

1. Gwich'in territory extends across the NWT/Yukon border and all the way into Alaska. Ernest's story tells of a few of his travels across colonial borders on these lands.
2. NorthMart is a chain of stores across the Canadian North, and it is often the only store in a community. You can purchase food, household goods, and outdoor supplies. The chain was created out of the legacy of the Hudson's Bay Company and is today based on an exploitative profit model. See Kristin Burnett and Travis Hay (2023) *Plundering the North: A History of Settler Colonialism, Corporate Welfare, and Food Insecurity,* Winnipeg: University of Manitoba Press.
3. Midway Lake Music Festival is held annually at Midway Lake along the Dempster Highway. It's a popular summer gathering for the region with fiddle music, drum dancing, square dancing, jigging, canoe races, fun, and camaraderie. It started in 1986 as a drug and alcohol-free event.
4. Many NWT communities have spring festivals in March or April of each year. For example, Fort McPherson has the Peel River Jamboree each April.

Alice Vittrekwa

FORT MCPHERSON

How did I cope? It was so sudden because Ernest was scheduled for a minor surgery when he was diagnosed. I thought, "Oh my God, this can't be happening. It can't be real." Then I reminded myself that I shouldn't feel bad. He's the one who should feel bad. I prepared myself that Ernest would get angry while we're there. But not once did he get mad. He accepted everything. He mentioned to everyone he spoke with during that time, "I accept everything and leave it in God's hands."

When we got his appointment sheet, he said, "Gee, we're going to be away from home a long time, away from our grandchildren." I told Ernest that it's not going to be easy, but we prayed. When we pray, we have to leave our grandchildren and children in God's hands. I told him, "You're here to get well and let's not make plans. From when we awake, we don't know what's coming our way. There are things we'll be able to do, and things we can't. But tomorrow is going to be another day." We continue to this day not making plans. That's a positive outcome from this situation.

It was difficult being away from home. During those times, someone always called me from home with words of encouragement or to ask if we need anything. All we requested from people was their prayers.

Photo by Tony Devlin.

Ernest did get sick and ended up in the hospital. I can remember waiting at Cross Cancer with him, and he was in pain. Then we had to go to the emergency room at the Royal Alex. In total we waited sixteen hours to find out the cause of his pain. There was a high chance that Ernest may have needed surgery in the night, but the doctor sent me back to Larga to rest. I was beat. At times I thought Ernest was sicker than they were telling us. I prayed for me and my family for strength so that we may cope with it.

There were bad days. One thing through those times is Ernest never let it affect his mood. One day I remember that Ernest yelled at me for his medication. He later apologized and told me that he really needed his pain medication right away. I said it's okay, and I reminded him that he was doing so well. He has his faith. He prays for everything and leaves it in God's hands. Cancer is something I wouldn't want to go through, but I do try to put myself in their shoes, the shoes of anyone who had cancer. I wonder how I'd feel to be told you have cancer. Not a good feeling! With him dealing with it in a positive way, it really helped me to be by his side. And that's what I can do is be there and ask God to be with him.

We knew people were praying for us; they were even fundraising for us. People showed us their support in their own way. Louisa Kay recorded a tape of requests sent to us on our little community radio station, CBQM, and sent it to us. I listened to this tape and all the messages, and I was so thankful to Louisa for this. I still have this cassette tape. People all showed up in their own way. They did anything and everything to comfort us. When we returned home, so much traditional food was provided to us by everyone. The young hunters were dropping meat off. Ernest's illness affected the younger generation of our community too. This one young boy dropped off a rabbit he hunted for Ernest; it was still warm when he brought it. All this really helped us.

I know lots of others are suffering with cancer. There's lots of people suffering, and we had lots of friends who we met through cancer. Some of them have passed away. When we travel on medical, we are often told that someone we know has passed away from cancer. Many of those who passed away did go through treatment. I realize that some patients are diagnosed with cancer too late. Yet other lives get prolonged with treatment. And for some patients, cancer returns again! I prepared myself for the reality that Ernest will get the help he needs for his illness, or not. I prepared myself as a mother, thinking of the effects it will have on our children and grandchildren. I had to keep telling myself that I had to be strong. It's because of the word Ernest uses, determination. He says, "I have determination to live, and my grandchildren are my medicine. They are the ones who keep me going by the help of God." Ernest has faith and knows his prayers are answered. I was once told that you get strength from pain. I said, how in the world could you get strength from pain? 'Cause when you're in pain that's all you're focused on is that pain. But I learned since that positive does come from that pain. With your experience you go through not only with cancer, you gain your strength. This helps you to help others who are going through similar situations. I'm grateful for my family who strongly supported me. Through the help of God, they were there.

What really helped me was all my family kept in daily contact with us to keep updated on Ernest's condition. They helped us financially during this time. At times they gave us traditional foods. These things that people did for us made me a stronger person. I used to let others' negative behaviour affect me. I prayed and asked God to help me with that, and he did! Now when situations arise, I'm able to calmly get through it. From that day we were told the sad news that Ernest has cancer to now, all that has happened has helped me to be a stronger person. This was my outcome.

To anybody who is diagnosed with cancer, I know it's painful to accept. You feel like you want to be alone and not let anyone know, stay in it alone. Eventually you will have to talk about it and let someone know. Don't hold it and don't think nobody cares or feel like no one can help or heal you. It's very easy to become angry or fall into addictions during these times of depression. Before all this happens, it's very important to know that sure, the cancer is going to be there — but there's hope. Some people live fourteen, fifteen years. But the most important thing is to talk about this illness. Talking is not going to take your cancer away, but the medicine could. The medical treatments like chemotherapy and radiation will help take away your cancer, and talking openly and honestly with another person helps your recovery towards being cancer free.

Maria Ellen Voudrach (Peterson)

FORT MCPHERSON

I am originally from Fort McPherson. I am the eldest daughter to Diane E. Koe and Danny Peterson; granddaughter to the late Albert Peterson and the late Florence Peterson and the late Thomas Koe and Eileen M. Koe. I am the wife to Bradley Voudrach of Tuktoyaktuk and we live together in Inuvik.

In September 2019, I found a lump on my breast and immediately went to the hospital in Inuvik. The lump, it didn't feel normal, it felt concerning, and immediately I felt scared so I got it checked out. The doctors reassured me that it was nothing to worry about but they made a referral for me to get a mammogram done. Finally, on November 19, of that year I had a mammogram and biopsy done in Yellowknife. On November 29 I was called back to the hospital. I didn't think much of it because I was reassured that it was nothing to worry about but that day, I was diagnosed with breast cancer. They were right in a way, the lumps I did find weren't cancerous but when I got the mammogram done, they found a cancerous lump way in the back of my breast, something I wouldn't have felt.

Maria Ellen Voudrach, her jijuu, and her baby Brielle.

I felt really scared and shocked, I was worried and had a lot of questions. But at that time, they couldn't answer any of my questions. I automatically thought, "Do I have weeks or months to live?" It was probably the scariest thing I've been through in my life. My mind was going crazy, and my heart was broken for my husband and loved ones.

My husband was with me at the time I was diagnosed. It was very hard on both of us as we were both in shock. I immediately called my grandmother Eileen to inform her, and she reassured me that things will be ok and to leave it in God's hands. Just a week before that, my grandfather Thomas was also diagnosed with prostate cancer, so this was even more devastating news for my family. I immediately went to Fort McPherson to be with family as I needed them the most at that time.

I received support from my family, friends, church family, and pretty much everyone in the Beaufort Delta. Anyone I had come across always gave me encouraging words; I also had people calling and sending me messages. It was really uplifting, and I can never thank them all enough as they gave me so much strength to keep fighting. I also had some ladies who had breast cancer who would reach out to me and provide their support and answer any questions I had, which was so helpful. There was support from everyone. We had people we were able to talk to. The NWT cancer navigators in Yellowknife were very helpful as well, and they provided a lot of support and resources, which made things so much easier.

When I was going through treatment, depression was bad, along with anxiety. I tried doing things that made me happy which was helpful; otherwise, my depression would have gotten worse. Hair loss during chemo was hard on me but I received support from family and friends who also shaved their hair in support of me. I was happy for that, and it made me stronger. I'd also say having cancer during the pandemic was hard in so many ways. Travelling back and forth from Alberta during that time was scary and stressful. I had to isolate three times that year. I couldn't see my family as much as I wanted due to restrictions that were in place for our safety.

Chemo was the toughest of it all. I had four rounds of chemo all together. The first two rounds were the toughest. I wanted to give up but my husband, my nieces and nephews, and other loved ones encouraged me to keep going. My grandfather passed away just before my third round so that gave me strength to keep pushing and keep fighting — I did it for him.

Things were a lot easier through my employment benefits. My husband came to every appointment with me. I can't even thank my husband enough for all he did for me during my cancer treatment. He helped me when I was so sick from chemo; he stayed by my side every second helping me with everything. He was also there when I got my surgery done, which was scary but again, he was there every step of the way helping me and encouraging me on a daily basis. Having an escort was very helpful and I can't even imagine having to do it alone. It's tough and I recommend having an escort as it is overwhelming with the information you receive and places you need to go.

Cancer has changed a lot for my husband and me. I'd say my faith has grown stronger; my husband and I attend church every Sunday if possible. We try to live a healthier lifestyle by eating healthier and exercising on a daily basis. I also have a different outlook on life now. I try not to stress over the little things and just try to live a better and happier life. We are more cautious with a lot of things now. I also have a lot of people come to me asking me questions because they have concerns of their own. I always encourage them to get it checked and always get a second opinion if they need it.

I also want to encourage all to get checked on a regular basis. If you are feeling ill and have concerns, please go see a doctor or nurse. Don't be shy, don't be scared, and don't ever feel like a bother: you have every right. Also please check on your loved ones, parents, grandparents, elders and if they have concerns, help them. Take them to see a doctor or nurse too.

I would encourage others facing cancer not to think the worst. I would comfort them and pray with them as that helped me a lot during my journey. I would also provide them with some of the resources I have received and just let them know they are never alone. Prayer is strong: it can get you through anything. Keep your faith strong and believe that the Lord will answer your prayers. Pray for others as it helps in so many ways. I truly believe I am here today because of prayers and my faith. Five years later, I have a daughter. I thought cancer took that chance away from me, but I have now been blessed with my miracle baby Brielle.

Charlie Furlong

AKLAVIK

I'm from Aklavik. My parents are Art and Ruth Furlong. My grandparents are Joseph and Bella Stewart on my mother's side. My grandparents on my father's side are Rosemary Clement and Art Furlong from the Sahtu Region. I grew up in Aklavik in a big family. We had a lot of get-togethers. We are a pretty close family. Through my grandmother I have a lot of relatives in Fort McPherson and Tsiigehtchic. I'm related to the Firths. I married Florence Blake of Fort McPherson; we have seven children, and I'm still here today.

All my life I had a pretty close bond with my grandparents. When I was born, my mother had tuberculosis. She was in the hospital for four years, so my grandparents took me in and raised me. I never really got to know my mother because of that.

I learned to speak my Gwich'in language and learned to understand the Gwich'in culture and traditions even though I had to go to the Roman Catholic mission school when I was young. I didn't stay there too long though. I was taken out of the mission and put in federal day school in Aklavik. Then in 1962 I went to high school in Inuvik.

After high school, in 1972, I was hired to work on the Berger Inquiry. I worked there for a number of years as the regional coordinator of the Mackenzie Delta Region. Then I worked for Dene Nation and the Métis Nation. I also worked in the Delta when we began the Mackenzie Regional Council, which is now known as the Gwich'in Tribal Council.

I was the first president of the Gwich'in Tribal Council. It was a good challenge. There were many arguments with Dene Nation and Métis Nation about land claims. In 1990, the Mackenzie Delta went on their own and negotiated a land claim with the government. I was one of the negotiators. I worked there pretty much up until my retirement.

Throughout my life I've had a lot of exposure to drugs and alcohol. I became an alcoholic. It really affected my life. In 1992, after we signed the Gwich'in land claim,[1] I went to treatment and quit drinking. I haven't had a drink since that time, but alcohol never leaves you. It affects your mind and body.

In my family there's lots of cancer. When I was 10 years old, I lost my granddad to cancer. My mother had breast cancer. My sister Rita had breast cancer. My daughter Annalee got breast cancer. All my aunties died of cancer. So, it's something you learn to live with. Every time I hear one of my relatives or friends is going to Edmonton for a check-up, I always wonder if they are going to come back with a cancer diagnosis.

Our community nurse, Rachel, is well liked within our community. She regularly monitored my bloodwork because of my family history of cancer. She noticed that something was wrong and wanted to do further testing. I went to Inuvik for a scope procedure of my colon. A few days later, Rachel called me and said that I had a spot of colon cancer the size of a loonie that was growing.

It was hard for me to tell my family I had cancer, especially my children and grandchildren, but they gave me strength to get through. It was for them that I tried hard. It was hard too because at that time my mother was dying of breast cancer. She was just two rooms down the hall from me in the hospital. My sister Rita told me to tell my mother, because I wasn't going to tell her. But my mother already kind of knew something was wrong so I told her. She felt bad, but she said, "Just listen to your doctor."

I went to Yellowknife to have it removed. Now I have half a colon and half a kidney too. There were other spots, and they didn't want it spreading so I began chemo. My operation was in April and my chemo began in July. I had to wait that long but I'm here today.

After samples were taken, it was confirmed that I was in the third stage. Now I know that cancer has four stages. Stage 1 and 2, you can deal with it by taking pills. Stage 3 you have to do chemotherapy or radiation. I did six months of chemotherapy. It was really hard on me. I lost a lot of weight. I even lost my ability to walk around. I couldn't do anything like I used to after chemo. I couldn't work or hunt. My whole system was out of whack. In the third month of chemotherapy, I told my partner Joanne that I couldn't take it anymore. She kept encouraging me, "Only three more months." I felt like giving up but then I would think about my family. I would think about my grandchildren, my girls, and my two sons. So, I just kept going. It's not easy. I can see why some people have a hard time, especially children. Even though I was sick I still tried to be a good example.

My family was there for me right from day one. My friends and the people that I worked with were there for me too. When I was in Yellowknife at Stanton Hospital for the operation that would remove my colon, the staff had to tell people to leave because there were too many visitors. That kind of support is really good. All the way through. In Edmonton it was the same thing. Everybody living there from up North used to come by. That felt good. People would bring me food — but the one thing I got tired of was caribou broth.

I was still going to the doctors during that time, getting check-ups and scans. Then in 2013 I started getting symptoms again. The doctor collected more tests and more samples. This time I had stage 4 prostate cancer. The doctor told me straight that it was too far advanced and that there was not much they could do. He said they would try to treat it with chemotherapy and radiation together.

While in Edmonton during that time, the doctor called me back to the Cross Cancer Institute and told me that they just got a new drug from the states to be used as a clinical trial. It was a long shot, but I was willing to try it. He said that all my bloodwork showed my system was good enough for the treatment. I said, "Sure, what do I have to lose?" I started that treatment in 2013. At that time the doctor said I would only have two years to live. He said not too many people go beyond two years with that stage of cancer, but here I am in my eighth year. A lot of people had faith in me. They kept me in their prayers. Lots of people were calling me all the time. They helped me to stay strong. That's one thing I learned about prayer: it works. If you believe in something hard enough, it's going to work. The good Lord isn't finished with me yet.

While I was going through that treatment, the Lord wanted to give me another challenge. I started getting sick again. They did more tests and found out I had cancer in my kidney. So, I had to return to Cross Cancer Institute in Edmonton again. The doctors told me it was also too far advanced so they cut my kidney out.

Just this January, the doctor reminded me of the two-year mark that they gave me. He said, "It looks like the drug is working." I don't have to go back to the Cross Cancer Institute anymore. I used to have to go every three months. They would put a needle into my stomach to get medicine into me. Now all they do is send the medication here to the Aklavik Health Centre and it is administered there.

Right now, I'm living with cancer but it's under control. I don't know how long it's going to last. I know it's there but I feel good. I do a lot of things. I work around the house. I'm getting my strength back. For me, cancer is something that is hard to live with but once I started learning more about it, I taught myself to live with cancer. What really concerns me is my family members. A lot of them feel bad for me. I give them material to look at to understand but it's still hard on them. They worry and that's hard on a person. There is lots of stress.

The thing you have to do with cancer is be open. If my story can help someone else then I will share it. I get invited to government workshops to speak about cancer. Afterwards I have people approaching me saying, "I'm going through the same thing." I tell them to keep going and don't look back. Through cancer I got to meet a lot of people. Some who are survivors and some who are living with it like me. We open up to each other. I get phone calls and tell people that they can call me any time, night or day. If I can help in any way I will.

My family expects me to beat cancer, and I tell myself that I'm not going to let them down. Sometimes I get so sick that I just want to give up, but thankfully that is just a passing thought. I rest a bit then when I wake up, I say to myself, "No. I have too many people thinking of me and praying for me." Even the church ministers and bishop were visiting me in Yellowknife while I was in the hospital. One time even the Legislative Assembly members all came to the hospital. I was lying there and next thing I knew they were all standing there in front of me. That kind of support helps you get through. I know that the sickness is going to be really bad for four or five days after chemo. After that I'm good again for about ten days until I have to go back for my next chemo. I know it will pass. I know what to expect now. I just wait it out.

After the third month of chemo and radiation my hair began thinning. I asked the nurse one morning, "Do you have a barber here?" I wanted to cut all my hair off. "No," she said. I didn't lose all my hair but there were some people in the hospital with me that were really self-conscious about it, especially women; they really don't like to lose their hair. It reminded me of mission school where everyone had to wear hats. Elders from Fort McPherson, Jane Charlie and Mary Teya, would send me jars of spruce gum and spruce juice. So I used to take that. I told my doctor that I was taking it, and he told me I could take whatever I felt was going to help me. I found out that some people refused to take conventional medicine like chemotherapy. They said they'd take traditional medicine only.

A lot of medicine is in your mind. You have to believe in it. So that's what I did. I don't know if it was the spruce gum that worked or the chemo that worked or both, but I know something worked. I'm sitting here today. It's been eleven years that I've been living with cancer. Depending on what type of cancer you have, there's all kinds of medicine out there.

If it is believed you might have cancer the doctors will run tests and do a biopsy. If you live in a small community, you will have to travel to Yellowknife and possibly Edmonton, where most of all the tests have to happen. If you have cancer that is where you will most likely find out what type of cancer you have. Then the doctor will tell you what treatment plan you will need. If you have a family, you have to remain strong for them. Even though you feel like nobody cares in the world, people do care. I thought that people would give up on me after a couple of months, but they stuck by me. That's very important. Some people in the community don't have anybody. I really feel for them so that's something that our leaders need to work on is to have people available to be by their side. Sometimes I've seen patients with no one with them when they are on medical travel. You have to have someone with you as an escort on medical appointments. You have to have someone who understands the disease. My partner Joanne asked the doctors a lot of questions. She knew what I was going to go through. She was my escort all the way through my sickness. I became an Elder during that time. Cancer patients shouldn't go without an escort. Lots of times when you're so sick, you can't hear what the doctor is saying. You need someone who understands. Cancer patients should never travel alone.

I've been involved in cancer awareness workshops. I speak to people all the way up the river. As a matter of fact, I worked for the government and facilitated workshops all the way down the valley talking about cancer. I think people are more aware but there's still a lot of work to do. We've got to get to the young people. They're the ones who find out when it's too late. Many have passed away because it was too late. There's still a lot of work to do, and a lot of information out there on cancer awareness that needs to be provided to Northerners. The Cross Cancer has a library of literature and videos that are available upon request. I took some when I came back one time, and I left them at the health centre in Aklavik to share. We have to keep moving, providing more information.

We've got a long way to go. We've got to keep at it. Talk to your leaders; they have to be involved. Part of working for your community is also working towards ensuring people are healthier. The government has to create positions in the regions, we need cancer navigators in the communities too. We need to train some of the nurses, but it's hard because they are in and out of our communities due to their contracts. It's not good when people only go to the nurse when they get sick; they should be getting regular check-ups. My family gets tested regularly. There should be more cancer prevention. I see some people who have had cancer and when it's cured, they don't change their unhealthy habits.

I always try to make myself available when I hear someone in the community has cancer. When Ernest Firth got sick from cancer, he didn't want to see anybody. But I called him, and he was happy to talk with me. We didn't talk about cancer, we just talked about growing up together and had a good long chat. I phoned Stephen Frost one morning because I knew Elders always get up early, and he was glad I called. We just talked and he told me this is probably the last time we'll talk. Sure enough, he passed away after that from cancer but just for that little while he was happy and that's the best medicine.

Note

1   The land claim is the Gwich'in Comprehensive Land Claim Agreement (GCLCA). The Gwich'in are represented by the Gwich'in Tribal Council (GTC), and the communities of Inuvik, Aklavik, Fort McPherson and Tsiigehtchic are identified as Gwich'in communities under the GCLCA. Read more about the GCLCA on the Gwich'in Tribal Council website.

Kirsten Fleuty

INUVIK

I have to look at this as a journey with funny stories; otherwise, I may cry continuously. I was diagnosed February 27, 2017, at the age of 52. I was told I had ductal carcinoma in situ (DCIS), stage 0, grade 3, right breast. No one in my immediate family had breast cancer; only distant cousins did. As I found out, DCIS is a presence of abnormal cells inside a milk duct in the breast. This is the earliest form of breast cancer. DCIS is non-invasive, which means it has not spread out of the milk duct. I am a lucky one as it was caught so early. I had no unusual lumps. I had a mastectomy with reconstructive surgery. The reconstructive part of the surgery procedure used tissue from the abdomen (skin, fat, and blood vessels) and moved it up to my right breast. Hence, I have a right breast full of my tummy fat. So, when I gain weight so does my breast.

When I was diagnosed, everything happened very fast. The appointments were made for me, an appointment every two weeks. I wish I could have collected Air Miles; I may have gotten a few free trips out of all this travelling to Yellowknife and Edmonton. It is amazing how I remember dates and certain experiences. Of course, there were many ups and downs along this journey, and all the feelings. On certain dates, I am not myself; those dates are when I was diagnosed, and my little surgery date, as I call it. Once, having a conversation with my plastic surgeon, I said, "my little surgery." He said, "That was no little surgery." My reply was, "I know but that is how I break it down for me. Who wants to hear that it was a seven-and-a-half-hour surgery with breast reconstruction?"

In November 2016, I had my regular mammogram. I went for the follow up on the mammogram and the young doctor said he wanted me to go to Yellowknife for a second mammogram and an ultrasound. I had "no worries." I had called medical travel to inform them I would be away over Christmas and could I have my appointment in January. The young doctor called me during Christmas to check if I knew when my appointment was. This was a first. I felt like the doctor really cared for me and wanted to make sure I had the appointment set. I went to Yellowknife with "no worries," because Inuvik did not have an ultrasound technician at the time. I was never worried. One week to the day, the young doctor called me to inform me that he is going to send me to Edmonton for a biopsy. I still had "no worries." The young doctor could not see me that week, and I went to another doctor but was not really informed about what the mammogram and ultrasound results were. I was worried about the dense breasts though no one explained to me what the calcifications meant in my breasts, nor even what to expect in a biopsy. Everything happens so fast.

I went to Edmonton two weeks later, on February 15, for the biopsy. Two weeks later, on February 27, I received the test results and was told I had DCIS. I did call my twin sister to tell her, but I kept it a secret for a few days from my children and family. The doctor in Inuvik made arrangement for me to meet a general surgeon in Edmonton two weeks later. I brought an entourage to the appointment: my daughter, twin sister, and mother. The doctor saw me first, and we talked about a lumpectomy and that the DCIS was about 3 cm long. I was comfortable with that, though he kept leaving the office to review the x-rays. The general surgeon kept asking me if I smoked, three times. The final time he asked, I said, "Should I start now?"

He also said, "Do not look on the internet." But I did look on the internet; this helped me with questions every time I met the doctors and even before the surgeries. Write all your questions down on sticky notes to give to the surgeon. I had a binder with all my personal information in it because I was asked the same questions over and over again. This way I did not have to remember the answers; I just gave them the binder.

The binder has everything in it — diseases, family medical history, any medications, a calendar for writing appointment dates, the sticky notes with the answers on them, etc. I also got copies of my pathologist reports. This was important because I never saw an oncologist, nor did I go to Cross Cancer after my initial surgery.

I was back in Edmonton at the Cross Cancer for a second biopsy in March. So off I go. Then I called the doctor's office on April 5 to say I am in Edmonton visiting if they need to see me. I get the phone call a half hour later asking if I could come in at 11:45 a.m. That day was the day I found out my lumpectomy (3 cm) became a mastectomy (7 cm). I did not want a mastectomy, as I had previously said to the general surgeon. This was a very upsetting day for me. I had meetings with the plastic surgeon about breast reconstruction later that week as well. The plastic surgeon was so funny. He drew on my chest to see where he would cut, talked a bit about the general surgeon and what he wanted in the surgery. Then all of a sudden, he says, "He makes his letters too wordy; he does not get to the point. He is asking two different things. I will need to talk to him." The plastic surgeon was walking out the door, but pops his head back into the room and asks, "Do you mind if I take a picture on my phone of your chest to text to the general surgeon to see if this is what he wants?" That made me laugh.

The following week, April 17, I had a CT scan. When you have that they warn you that you may want to go to the bathroom. I can say, yes, that actually is the feeling you have in this procedure. Same day another consultation with the plastic surgeon and more information about what the procedure is. On that day, when I met with the plastic surgeon he just had come out of surgery, and he apologized that he was in scrubs. He also indicated he had torn his very colourful socks. My friend came with me that day and we had a laugh. We wondered if he darned his own socks and if he did, what kind of stitch did he do to fix them?

Back in Inuvik, the two weeks flew by, and on April 27, I had not received my medical travel information even though I was leaving that day. I usually got the information three days before I travel, but this time, I did not. This was very stressful for an already stressful situation. In the morning, I emailed I had not received my travel information, and I had a pre-op appointment in Edmonton the next day at 7:30 a.m. and that I could not miss this appointment as I was having a very serious surgery. I finally received all the information by 10:30 a.m. and I was heading to the airport at 11:30. When medical travel books your flights, you are leaving the next day after your appointment. I was in the hospital for seven days after my surgery; therefore, I would not have made the flight the next day. I learned I can change my return flights after my surgeries.

At the pre-op appointment the nurse was asking all the same questions that I had in my binder. This was very helpful because I did not have to try to remember all the little details about my life. The nurse called my doctors the "dream team," and they certainly were dreamy to look at during each consultation and even when going under. I know that she meant that these doctors are considered a very good team for mastectomy and reconstructive surgery. It made me laugh, and I figured I was in good hands, literally.

On May 1, the plastic surgeon did his markings on my breast for where he was going to cut me. He gave me a black permanent marker and asked for me to bring it back as he loses them all the time. This made me laugh. Later I bought him a gift of black sharpies and put labels with his name on it so he would not lose them anymore. I also went and got the dye injected in my breast to see where my lymph nodes are. It was a busy day before surgery.

May 2 is my son's birthday. I did not get to choose the day, the surgeons do. I still apologize to my son about my surgery day. The day of surgery I was up very early. I showered and re-drew the markings. Plus, I added a little extra drawing above his markings, a skull and crossbones. The doctor said he did not see my markings until the very end of surgery when he was undraping me. I asked him to look after the taa-taas and then I do not remember anything after that.

After surgery, for the first forty-eight hours, the specially trained nurses woke me up every hour to check the blood vessels using a doppler, then every two hours and finally every four hours over the six days. This is exhausting and I was very tired. The best part was I had my very own private nurse for three days, then I had to share them with other patients. While listening to the blood vessels the nurses also check to make sure my skin is not turning black, which means the skin is dying. Well, I did have a small little patch of dying skin. So, a new worry while in the hospital. Along with that, I had to get two pints of blood as I am anaemic. I have never had a blood transfusion before, and it was a bit worrying — one more thing to add to my adventures of having a mastectomy.

When I left the hospital, I did have home care come to my mom's house to help and she gave instructions and brought various items to help with the black spot. I had to change the bandages every day. I slept on my mother's couch recliner for six weeks. The first few weeks I could hardly lift my body off the recliner and needed help. My brother and sister-in-law were there for a week, and my nephew came another time for a weekend. All I needed was to have an arm support in front of me so I could use it to help lift myself off the couch. I of course have many funny stories. Like one night my brother went down to where his wife was sleeping and during the night I had to really go to the bathroom. I called my brother, he did not hear me; I called his cell phone, he did not answer. I finally call the house phone and he picked up. Could he come to help me get out off the couch and then he can go back to bed?

When my brother left, then my mom and I had a few days by ourselves. I needed a bit of help changing the bandages. My mom was so funny. So, we were changing my bandages, and my mom would put on the gloves, then she would touch the bed with her hands to help her walk around. I would say "You have to change your gloves, Mom." She did this three times, taking them off and changing them because she touched something. So, we worked out a plan so that it would not be a fifth time. That was when I called my nephew to bring up a chair for Grandma. She would sit beside me to help change the bandages. My mum put on her gloves, then put up her hands and said, "I saw this in a movie once." She did not want to touch the bed with the gloves on again. We laughed so hard; it was a great belly laugh, and we needed that.

My twin sister never left the hospital when I had all my surgeries. She'd help out during the day also and came to every appointment except one. She suggested the binder with dividers to put all the information in order, for example, your own medical history before your cancer diagnoses. She also suggested to have someone to write everything down when you are with all your doctors. She said, "What I hear and what you hear could be two different things. You get blasted with so much information and so many decisions it helps you figure things out." I learned that it's ok to ask the same questions over and over again. It may not change the answer, but it did give me peace of mind. Sometimes you may not remember that you already asked the questions, because everything happens so fast.

I had to go for another surgery as they did not get enough of the margins as per the pathologist report. The margins are something you do not want to hear about. This was also when I learned from the pathologist report that the 7 cm was actually 14 cm, thus I had to have the mastectomy. I believe I am like the 5 percent of DCIS patients who have to have a mastectomy because of all the calcifications inside the ducts.

I have had several plastic surgeries to make sure everything looks correct. My right breast will never be the same; it does not look the same and does not have any feeling. That is my reality. I did have the plastic surgeon create a nipple for me and have a nipple tattoo. In one of my appointments with the plastic surgeon, he was touching my breast and said, "Yes they do feel about the same," moving his hands feeling the weight of them. I laughed because no one has ever touched my breast and made that comment before. Another time he walked in on me while I was changing out of my clothes for an appointment. I had just bought a very sexy new bra, and he saw it. The nurse came in an apologized but said "I will be teased all day for this." I laughed and told the nurse no problem; I have my new sexy bra on, and it was as if I was wearing a bikini. We laughed together at that.

There are still worries at the back of my mind; every little ache, pain, or not feeling well makes me worried, "Do I have cancer again? Where did it spread? Do I need to go to the doctor?" The radiologist said, "There were no floaties so not to worry about it," but in my mind it is a worry. I have recently found a lump on my right breast that is a bit worrisome. I also have a thickness in my uterus, which was found as a side note when I thought I was having an appendix attack. I am only four years from my initial diagnosis. The statistics are another challenge for me. I am overweight and trying desperately to lose the weight, but I find this very difficult. This can lead to my life being short. I want to live to 100!

I have laughed and cried. I have not so much asked, "Why me?" I accepted that I had breast cancer, that it is a fact of life. My dad had various cancers, my mom just recently, and my older sister, too. These cancers are kind of related. I did not have radiation or chemo. It was caught early but it is always at the back of my mind. That is my reality.

Inuvik has a wonderful cancer support group, which includes all different kinds of cancer. We call it "Our Group" and I can say I have been privileged to be a part of the group right from the beginning. Our Group has gracious leaders, and everyone is welcome. Today, I continue to tell people to get a mammogram. I tell about the upsides: my funny stories about my doctors and Mom. I make people laugh. As I was travelling down to Edmonton from Inuvik, I was talking, and a person said to me I should be a comedian because I made him laugh over everything little thing that had happened to me. I said to him that it was a select audience who would know what I was talking about.

One needs laughter, conversations, and enjoyment. I hope this helps you with your journey, and knowing others may have had similar experiences as you. No one tells you what to really expect but keep asking those questions. Remember, your own hope, joy, and laugher will help.

Since this was written my mother passed away, and I would like to dedicate this to her. My mom, Crystal, was with me throughout this journey. She taught me to be strong and independent, and to never give up. I would also like to thank my family and friends for their support too. "Life is good," as Mom would say.

Sandra Lynn Malcolm

INUVIK

My husband David's journey with cancer began in May 2015, long before anybody knew he was ill. David and I were walking the bypass road together in our community of Inuvik. The walk is seven and a half kilometres, a beautiful route that took us approximately one hour and twenty minutes to complete. It was a wonderful way to release the stress of the day and reconnect with each other. The walk took us from a relatively flat stretch to an incline in the hills to the north of Inuvik. We walked the route daily beginning in the spring of 2014.

One Friday evening after dinner, as we walked the bypass road, I elected that we take the route with the long climb. We were about two thirds of the way when David said, "You know, Sandra, I'm not sure if I should tell you this, but I've got a pain in my heart." I went into high alert. David was a 75-year-old overweight Caucasian male. His dad died around the same age of a massive heart attack. David walked the rest of the way even though I suggested calling a cab to get to the hospital. We went to the emergency room. When we saw the doctor he said, "We don't know what it could be. It's not your heart. The blood test shows no stress on your heart. Just go home and take it easy for a while." So, David and I went home and carried on with our normal lives, including walking the bypass road daily.

Sandra Lynn's and David Malcolm's hands.

When summer was over and the temperature dropped to -15, I had long gotten over my cough from the flu we caught on our trip to Anchorage, Alaska. We had gone on a yearly Christian retreat there in July. But David's cough didn't go away; instead, it morphed into a dry cough. I said, "David you're still coughing? Something is wrong!" He said, "No, I just have an itch in my throat. Must be the dry air." A month later I said again, "David, you're still coughing." He would reply, "Sandra, you're starting to nag." So, I stopped talking to him about it because I did not want to upset him, but it continued to worry me.

Then on November 26, 2015, David brought lunch to my work, and as I watched him walk across the parking lot I thought, "Goodness, he's walking really slowly." I ran downstairs and got my sandwich from him. Later that evening he told me that on his walk home he suddenly felt faint and had to stop and rest to catch his breath, and when he got home, he had a nap. My heart leaped into my throat. "We're going to the hospital," I said, and he agreed.

David told the doctor what had happened to him that afternoon. The doctor did some bloodwork and told David he needed a wheelchair. The results of the bloodwork showed that David's heart was stressed. He was to take a medevac to the cardiac unit at the Sturgeon Hospital north of Edmonton the next day. David stayed in the hospital that night while I went home and packed. I was anxious. I phoned my sister, Janice, and told her what was happening.

The next day I asked to be on the medevac, but medical travel would not allow it. I cried as I watched the paramedics unload David from the ambulance, wheel him over to the waiting jet and load him in, still strapped to the gurney. When the plane departed, I thought, "What do I do? How do I cope?"

I got into my vehicle. I was shaking as I started the car and drove back home. I could no longer hold my fear at bay. I was terrified. I called my mentor, Judy, and with her help I was able to make a plan. I would get on a flight to Edmonton whether or not I would be reimbursed for the cost. David needed me to be with him during medical appointments because of his hearing impairment. Later on, when the doctors became aware of David's severe hearing loss, I was able to accompany him as his non-medical escort.

When I got to Edmonton, I rented a car and drove to the Sturgeon Hospital and arrived there in the late evening. David was in the Intensive Care Unit in very good spirits. He told me they ran tests on his heart and that his heart was fine but something else was wrong. They began a series of tests to find out. David had a CT scan on Monday morning and another one that same afternoon. We heard nothing. The next day hospital staff came in to take David for another CT scan. More waiting. Later that day a physician came and told us the results of the CT scans. He had a large mass on his left kidney. "We're transferring you to the University Hospital in Edmonton. They'll treat the mass there," the doctor said. David wanted to delay the operation, but the doctor replied, "I'm surprised you're still alive. You could be dead in five or ten minutes." I felt like I had been hit by a semi-truck.

Before David's surgery, very aware that he might not survive the operation, I gave him a much-needed haircut. We were told that he had a 70 percent chance of dying on the operating table. It was a serious operation. There were only five surgeons in Canada who had the skills to do the operation. I ran alongside him as they pushed him into the operating room. We thanked each other for our wonderful thirty years together and said our good-byes, just in case.

The operation took six hours and David emerged successfully. The next day I called our naturopathic doctor in Yellowknife and told her a cancerous mass was found on David's left kidney. I asked her what we could do. She said we should wait until after the doctors began treatment, then she would prescribe natural remedies.

After the surgery, David was transferred to a private room. I requested a cot and spent at least 95 percent of the time with him in the room. I left only to get food from the hospital cafeteria. I went back to the hotel room about once a week to shower and change. In that private room, I could see David slowly healing.

As soon as he was able, David began accessing online medical journals. He found out that 80 percent of people who survived his operation were dead within six months. He began researching clear cell renal carcinoma (kidney cancer), nutrition, and naturopathic means of recovery from cancer. A study in the medical literature showed that sugar feeds cancer. When our bodies have an overload of sugar, our immune system, the very system in our bodies that fights cancer, shuts down. Refined sugar was an obvious culprit, but so were natural sugars such as honey, maple syrup and fruit juices. Foods that were digested quickly into sugar, high glycemic foods, were also a culprit. David began searching lists of foods, so we would know which ones were high glycemic. His kidney function was very poor, so he also researched what foods to avoid if one has kidney disease. I began scouring cookbooks to prepare tasty meals that would help heal David. Making vegetable-based meals in the Arctic, where fresh fruits and produce are often not available, was challenging.

As soon as David could walk, we resumed walking regularly. At first, we went very short distances. David's diagnosis shocked our families. It had come out of nowhere. I continue to be grateful for those who supported us. David was discharged ten days post-surgery, and we were scheduled to fly back to Inuvik the next morning. Back at home David's daughter Anne visited. I went back to work, and Anne stayed until mid-January.

By September of that year, I was very stressed and requested stress leave from work. I went home, got on the internet and booked flights and a hotel room to Fort Lauderdale, Florida. In no time, David and I were there. David sat by the pool and I walked for miles along the beach every day. Sand between your toes is a therapeutic approach to stress relief. I took ten days off work and then went back and resumed my full schedule.

David was scheduled for another CT scan in February at the Cross Cancer Institute in Edmonton. After the CT scan David was scheduled to meet with the oncologist, who would prepare us for David's chemotherapy treatment. However, the oncologist excitedly announced that David would not need chemotherapy because the CT scans showed a visible reduction in the size of cancerous nodes in his lungs and pulmonary cavity. What great news!

Life after that was relatively stable until July 2017, when we received the gut-wrenching results that the cancer was back. There were two tumours growing on David's spine. One on his tailbone and the other mid-back. David would get five radiation treatments followed by a chemotherapy treatment administered by pill at home.

While he was taking the chemo, David began experiencing a weird pain in his head and neck. A CT scan showed a tumour on the left side of his spine at the base of his skull. We spent Christmas with our family that year and got a dog to keep David company while I worked. David stopped chemo after two months when he said to me, "Sandra, I'd rather be dead than take more chemo." In tears, I agreed with him, "Yes, David, death would be better than this."

The doctor gave him another option, immunotherapy treatments, which, combined with the naturopathic medicine that he was already taking, extended his life four more years. We travelled to Edmonton every two weeks for immunotherapy treatments. My workplace supervisors supported me, and I found out that homecare was available; they began providing at-home nursing and physician care for David.

On November 30, 2020, David had a CT scan done. We got the results two weeks later. The oncologist told him, "Your cancer is growing. You have three to six months to live. You are now palliative. We are discontinuing all treatment and tests but will continue to prescribe pain medication to keep you comfortable." It was our pre-Christmas gut punch.

In January 2021, in together time, David said to me, "Sandra, I am ready to die." I agreed with him, "Yes, David, it is time. There is no other alternative for you, and I'm okay with you dying. But David, you need to know, I'm choosing life." David had a bad fall on March 6, 2021, and began bleeding from his head. He said to me, "I love you," and then slipped into a semi-conscious state from which he never re-awoke. Just after midnight on March 9, 2021, as I held him, he passed into eternity.

The months after remain a blur to me. I couldn't think, slept a lot, walked at least one hour per day, and sewed. I couldn't comprehend what I was reading; I couldn't fill in simple forms. Passive suicide — letting myself sleep and lie around until my body broke down completely — was what I wanted to do, but I had promised myself, David, and God that I was choosing life. So, I tried to grasp on to life. Three friends visited me regularly and I would walk to visit one couple. I also had a huge online support network. Gradually, my ability to think improved, I returned to work, and I began to experience a glimpse of stability and with it, hope.

David is gone now, and my life is changed forever. I miss my best friend, the person with whom I laughed, cried, dreamed, and schemed. Today, David is dwelling in the mansion promised by Jesus. The grieving journey is not easy. Since David died, I began to recognize a myriad of my character defects stemming from my human nature and the emotional pain that I absorbed in my journey of life. I believe that David was sent to me by God, as a helpmate to assist my emotional and spiritual growth. Now that David is gone, God is directing me to turn to Him in all things. I know that God is keeping me alive for a reason. I don't know what the reason is, and I don't need to. That's not my business, that's God's business. My business is to live each day to the fullest, accept the outcome and grow spiritually, always preparing for the time when I too will leave my mortal shell behind and dwell in one of the mansions in God's house.

Winston Moses

INUVIK

I was born down in the Yukon Territory at a place called Old Crow. I lived here and there and then finally settled down in Inuvik. I have my family here with me now. I don't think I'll be going anywhere else. I'll just stay here.

I thought about people who had gotten cancer, but I never really thought too much about what cancer was until one day I went down to see the doctor for an annual check-up. I looked up on the wall and saw a poster about getting tested for cancer if you are over fifty. My first thought was, "I don't think that is me," but I told the doctor I would like to get a test anyway and he said that was a wise decision. I took the test and here I am today. If I didn't, I'd probably be six feet under.

I had blood tests and all the other procedures you go through when you're diagnosed. They told me I had to go to Yellowknife, so I went and got more tests in Yellowknife. Then they said they were still not quite sure, so they had to do another test in Yellowknife.

Then one day they said they would have to send me back to Edmonton. I had already gone to Edmonton for tests and was being sent again. When I got back to Yellowknife from Edmonton the second time, instead of telling me what they found or asking me questions, they just sent me home

Photo by Tony Devlin.

because it was close to Christmas. My son, Alfred, was with me at the time. I asked him, "Why didn't they ask me or tell me anything?" He told me they couldn't do anything right now, so it was best to just go home and spend Christmas together.

About a month later someone called me and told me I had cancer. I couldn't believe it. I had been healthy most of my life. I felt a little bit afraid. I wondered how my kids would take it when I had to tell them. I had always been there for them. There would be no one there for them. I was afraid of how they were going to react to the news, so before I told them I talked to some people who had cancer and asked how they talked to their children. That helped me to share the news with them. I didn't know how the kids felt about it. I'm sure they talked amongst each other. My children are on their own now. We prayed. I'm sure a bunch of people prayed for me too.

I know I am going to die one day so I just thought to myself, "Deal with it the way you would like to deal with it," and I just kept up with the doctor's instructions so it did not increase more. If you follow what the doctor says, then maybe you will be okay. I always prayed that I do not want to die of cancer. A natural death would be okay. It is hard to go through something like this.

I had a few drinks here and there to take the cancer thoughts out of my mind and to ease the pain a little bit. I am glad that I knocked that off and stopped drinking. When you get a disease like cancer, it makes you think about how you have to get things done that you need to get done. I didn't want to leave things undone. I didn't want to ask myself, "How come you didn't say this? How come you did that?" I wanted to make amends.

They were gonna put a needle in my spine and in my lungs where I had cancer. They could see it on the screen. They told me that with this type of operation some people pull through and some don't. In my situation it was a difficult procedure because they would have to go through a main artery, but there was something in the way of the artery and it could somehow erupt. They did not want to take a chance on that happening so they said they would have to wait to do the procedure. Then the doctors called me back to Yellowknife and I thought, even if there is a danger with the operation, I will probably still go through with it. So, I said to my wife, "Let's go for it."

When we went into the doctor's office, they wanted me to see the x-ray. They showed me where the cancer had been on my lung and it was gone. It was clear. I jumped for joy.

Now I tell my relatives who have cancer my story and they feel a little better about it. I tell them that if you pray there is a chance for healing. I am very glad that I can tell others my story. Do not give up hope just because the doctors say you have cancer or that they can't cure cancer.

I'm so glad for the Inuvik Cancer Support Group because if not for them I would be at home feeling sorry for myself. When I found the group I thought, "These are people that care for us and make sure that we deal with cancer correctly." The group is a place where you can speak to other people and share together. Some people in the group might not have cancer themselves but they have loved ones who do.

Cancer affects everyone, not only the person who has it. It also affects their loved ones and friends too. When you have cancer, it feels like you have to put things in order. I felt like I had to leave some sort of money behind for an emergency, so I got in touch with social workers and they helped me. I asked them to help me look after things if I died and I felt a little better.

When someone is in distress of any kind, especially hearing the news that they have cancer, that kind of news can hurt. So before they say anything, I say, "Come in," and I give them a hug. Sometimes that's all they need until the words start flowing. I invite them in, have a cup of tea, and keep an eye on them. Some people just burst out crying and some of them sit down for a while and then eventually say, "I've got cancer." They come knocking at my door because they know I'm here to help, usually with words. I say, "It's okay for now." And I pray with them, and then I give them tea. It sinks in. They feel comfortable and no longer scared. Then they start talking about it. They want to know how it is to have cancer. I try to give them some kind of happiness and hope and throw in a few laughs too.

Laughing is medicine and so is crying. Don't ever say, "Don't cry," because holding sadness inside can make us sick. Make sure you go in for your regular check-ups. I would encourage those who have had cancer to approach people who have just been told they have cancer to help give them hope because words are powerful. Do not give up.

Don't think, "poor me," because you're just letting yourself down with negative thinking. Be grateful and help others because you're going to save someone. If you have cancer, don't be afraid.

I hope you all are reading this and enjoying a nice hot tea or coffee with sugar-free peanut butter fudge. Prayers for a blessed day everyone.

Ashley Wendland

INUVIK

I was 27 years old when I was diagnosed. I had moved to Inuvik from the East Coast in May 2017 to work and experience life in the Arctic.

It was four months after settling in Inuvik that I began to experience my cancer symptoms: blurred vision and the feeling of heaviness in my left eye. This is where the difficult part of what was to have been a beautiful, yet frigid, adventure started. A visit to the Inuvik Regional Hospital emergency room provided no diagnosis or relief from my symptoms.

The symptoms continued and forced me back to the ER a few days later. On this visit, I requested a referral to see a specialist, the nearest one being in Yellowknife. That appointment saw me leave with no answers or relief of symptoms. I was sent back to Inuvik with another referral to a different ophthalmologist in Edmonton at a later date.

After various types of testing in Edmonton it was determined that there was a lesion attached to my retina. I again was sent back to Inuvik with a referral to a third specialist at a later date back in Edmonton. My third trip out of Inuvik to a specialist confirmed the existence of a lesion sitting directly on my retina. Again, I was sent back home unsure of the situation with my eye and was scheduled for another follow-up appointment. During that time the specialist consulted with other experts. He knew what he was looking at was exceedingly rare and confusing to even him and he was one of the leading ocular surgeons in the country. My fourth trip back to the specialist resulted in yet more testing and imaging, but still no diagnosis. I was told to expect a call within a week, before the Christmas holiday.

The call and diagnosis came on December 28, 2017. I was diagnosed with ocular melanoma, specifically choroidal melanoma, a type of melanoma that occurs at a rate of approximately 6 in 1 million individuals per year. The day I received my diagnosis, I was lying in bed. The rest of my recollection is dark; I sort of blanked out. It was the coldest and darkest month of the year. I know she started talking about treatment; she had already sent me a schedule and booked me in for everything. All I had to do was book my medical travel. My only support was my husband and the doctors at the Inuvik Hospital. I was absolutely terrified for what was to come as the fear of my mortality set in.

After hearing the words, "You have cancer," the first person I called was my now ex-husband, Luke. He ran home to be with me and consoled me as I lay in bed. From there we went to speak to one of the doctors at the Inuvik Regional Hospital, and I said, "I need help. I've just been diagnosed. I don't have family here. What resources can I access?" The doctor prescribed me some medication for anxiety. Luke was by my side, but I still felt alone.

I called my mother next. She was trying to be positive for me, "We are going to get through it; there's nothing they can't fix." I thought, can't we be angry for a minute that it's cancer? I was only fixated on the scary, possible reality of losing my eye. Am I going to go blind? Am I going to lose my hair? Word spread fast among my family. Everyone was in shock and denial that their 27-year-old relative had been diagnosed with cancer, 8000 km away from them.

The initial treatment required the surgical placement of a radioactive plaque, a metal plate, on my eye. The plaque stayed attached, releasing radiation, for a period of five days. Many subsequent follow-up appointments and treatments were required. I didn't qualify for subsidies for flights or accommodation, given I am not First Nations or Inuit. Many times, I was denied an escort, as my follow-up visits were seen as routine. I fought hard, with the support of social workers at the Cross Cancer Institute, to obtain the right to have an escort. I was receiving chemo injections, leaving me partially blind for the duration of my time in Edmonton. At any time, my doctor could have told me cancer had returned. I would have been alone. I spoke to CBC News twice about the challenges of being a patient in the North as I felt I needed to be a voice for those who would struggle after me.

To support my mental health during and beyond treatment, I joined various ocular melanoma Facebook support groups. I joined Young Adult Cancer Canada and found Imerman Angels, which is an organization that provides one-on-one support to someone who has been through the same cancer diagnosis and can offer stories of hope. These groups were incredibly important to me, and they are still important to me on my cancer journey. I ended up connecting with a girl named Rachel who was diagnosed at the same time as me. She was living in Florida. We had treatment at the same time.

I also met a girl from Edmonton who had the same specialist as me. It was nice to speak to somebody who had already had the same treatment to see that life actually does go back to normal, albeit a different type of normal. She was already back to work, she was dating, and you couldn't tell that her eye had been through trauma.

I found it very hard to be away from my family. However, the people of Inuvik were happy to provide support by preparing meals, walking my dogs, and raising money for my medical travel. I will be forever grateful for these kind acts. I had people calling me to check in to see how I was doing. I had community members donating money so I could stay in Edmonton for as long as needed. I wouldn't have had that type of support if I hadn't lived in a community like Inuvik. The Inuvik Cancer Support Group was enjoyable, too. I didn't feel alone. It would have been good to have support offered to caretakers because they really deal with a lot. I know my mother and father still struggle with what happened.

Cancer was eye opening, so to speak. The minute I was diagnosed, the things I thought were important pre-cancer were no longer important. What was important to me was my happiness and I promised myself that if I survived cancer, I would make changes to ensure I lived a full, happy life. Now I'm living life on my terms.

I continue to receive second chances at life every time my annual scans tell me I am cancer free. When I go for my follow-ups, it's triggering. I'm very worried that when I go in, I'm going to hear bad news. I still have to do my yearly MRI and chest x-ray to make sure my primary tumour hasn't spread. I just hit my five-year cancerversary since my diagnosis and my last radiation was in February. When diagnosed with this type of cancer, there's a 50 percent chance it could spread to your liver within five years. I have been lucky it hasn't shown up anywhere else in my body.

I experience survivor's guilt. My friend Rachel, from Florida, has passed away. Her cancer spread to her liver quite quickly after it was diagnosed in her eye. We were diagnosed with the same cancer, at the same time, and we were almost the same age. When her mother wrote to me to tell me she passed away, I had no idea it had gotten as bad as it had. I felt guilty celebrating my five-year cancer-free milestone because at the time she was clearly going through something much more difficult.

Cancer has changed me. I am now living and working in Australia with my new partner. I am also giving back to the beautiful organizations that helped me through my diagnosis by writing blog posts and advocating for young adult cancer thrivers in the Northwest Territories and Canada. I preach about not only sunscreen and eye protection but getting your eyes tested and speaking up for yourself when faced with health challenges.

I used to feel that I didn't have control of the life I was living. Cancer changed that. Once I had healed physically from treatment, I pivoted and made changes I was never brave enough to make prior to my diagnosis. I left the profession I disliked to begin meaningful work with the Inuvialuit Regional Corporation[1] as a health promoter. I ended a marriage and eventually moved across the world. I'll never say that cancer was a blessing, but it did give me a kick in the butt to make a change. Now I don't even recognize the person I was during that time.

To anyone experiencing cancer: there is hope. Reach out for support if you are feeling alone or anxious. For me, the best thing I did was speak to other cancer patients. No amount of medication or talking to my mother, partner, or friends was as helpful as hearing from people who are going through the same thing, especially someone who has been through the same type of cancer. It's invaluable.

Note

1   The Inuvialuit Regional Corporation represents the collective interests of the Inuvialuit, with a goal to improve the well-being of the Inuvialuit. It was established in 1984 to manage the settlement outlined in the Inuvialuit Final Agreement: the first comprehensive land claim agreement signed north of the 60th parallel. See the Inuvialuit Regional Corporation website for more information.

Ruth Wright

INUVIK

I was born April 6, 1960, in Aklavik to Jane and Harley Wright. I'm the oldest in my family but I'm still treated like the baby. I first got introduced to cancer when I was about 10 years old. My little sister Ruby Ann was born, and within a year or two my auntie Rowena realized something was wrong. My auntie had adopted Ruby Ann when she was born so she lived most of her life in Old Crow and would only come here to see the doctor or for a visit. They finally sent her out to Edmonton and she was diagnosed with leukaemia. She would get really sick to the point where she was just lying on the couch. I couldn't figure out why the doctors couldn't just give her a pill and she'd be okay. I realized the sickness she had was cancer and it was inside her blood.

When she was about 6, she was on the back steps talking to our younger sister Elaine. I just happened to be walking past the open window when I overheard her say, "Well, I'm going to die pretty soon." Elaine was 4 years old and didn't realize what she meant. They were having a discussion between little sisters about how Ruby Ann was dying and going to see Jesus and everything would be alright; she's not going to have any pain. I couldn't believe it. I was sitting inside just sniffling away.

I would ask her, "What did they do to you when you went to Edmonton?" She would say, "Oh they gave me this medication, they gave me four milligrams of this stuff." She knew everything. She knew all the big, long words about her medication and treatment, and she was just a little kid. Goodness. When she passed, although it was really heart-breaking for someone so young to pass away, I knew in my heart that she knew she was going somewhere else.

When I was in grade 8, a classmate of mine, Donna Ross, passed away. Donna was one of those free loving spirits. That's the first time that I thought, besides my sister, who was born with it, "You could get cancer and it could just take you." For all her peers at school it was really life affecting because she was so young, and cancer came and took her. When she died, we didn't discuss cancer at all. If she was sick, she sure never told us. It was the 1970s and we didn't know much about it.

My stepdad Jerry got cancer in his bones. When he came North, he worked as a driller. He came into our life and was always a hard worker but then he got sick. It was strange to see him sick and on the couch. It was hard when he passed away because we were so used to him being around. He would say, "When I die, watch your mom." He quit drinking and really tried his best to get my mom to quit drinking too, but drinking was how she dealt with stress. He said, "Make sure the bills are paid and make sure she eats." My mom was lost after he passed on. He lived here for thirty years, and he would never ever eat muskrats. He tried to speak Gwich'in, but he couldn't pronounce lots of words. It was funny when he tried.

When he was in the hospital in Edmonton I went to visit him. That hospital had the longest hallways in the world. People were lined up in beds in those long hallways, that's how busy it was. When I got to his room there was just one man in there. It wasn't Jerry. This man had no mouth. He had cancer of the mouth. At first, I was kind of shocked, but I asked him if he knew my stepdad. I sat and talked to him while Jerry was out smoking. When Jerry came back, he was with another man who had throat cancer and had a big hole in his throat as a result. When he smoked, he would just hold the cigarette in front of his throat and breathe in. I was shocked again but then Jerry said, "He's only got a couple of weeks to live. Smoking is the one thing he's been doing since he was a teenager. How are you going to take that away from him?" I thought, "You're right. That's not my place to say anything."

Jerry ended up having his leg below his knee removed. When released from the hospital he came home, and everybody rallied around my mom to help her cope. Then a couple of months later, Jerry started getting sick again. He went to the local hospital and was sent back out to Edmonton, where they removed his other leg below the knee. He was sent home and just a couple months after that, he passed away. I could see the progression of the disease. I thought if the doctor could remove the cancer, then it's gone for good. But it was in Jerry's bones, and it moved around.

I didn't know my mom had cancer when I escorted her to Edmonton to deal with what I thought were ulcers. While they were doing tests on her, I went down the hallway and saw the doctor coming out of the room, so I asked what the results were. He said, "Well, she's got stage 4 colon cancer and I give her about three weeks to live." I was mad at him. How dare he tell me my mom's got three weeks to live. At the same time, I thought, "She's got three weeks to live, so we are going to make it the best we can." I went back to her room, and she asked if I saw the doctor because she saw me run by. I said, "Yes, I saw him," and asked her, "You knew?"

And she said, "Well, we thought it might be."

I said, "And you never told me? I always thought I was the brave one of the family."

"Well, I didn't want to tell you because I wanted you to be here with me," my mom replied.

I said, "Okay, I'm over being shocked so let's deal with this." I phoned Larga and they said the doctor had already called them. They tried to book us back home, but all the planes were full because it was near Christmas. I thought, "Oh my God, we are going to have to stay here for two weeks out of her three weeks to live." But Larga made a few calls, packed our stuff, and said they were able to get us on a medevac plane was travelling North. I cried. I was so thankful that my family could be with her.

When we got back to Inuvik she was admitted to the hospital, and it was a shock for everybody to hear of her diagnosis. All her friends would come to visit. After two weeks she was up and walking around. Even the doctor was surprised, and a little while later she got to go home. For a few weeks everything was okay, and I thought, "Wow that doctor down there doesn't know what he's talking about."

She quit drinking. She said, "I don't want my grandkids' last memory to be of me being drunk." After that, all the grandkids would come over every day to visit her. We would go down for walks to Twin Lakes. At that time Twin Lakes had nothing there, just a bunch of bushes. We used to go down there for picnics and look for leaves and rocks. We would take blankets, and my mom and her grandkids would sit around. It was really good. It went on and on over the summer, the fall, and the winter. She lived for three and a half years after her diagnosis. Thank goodness that she was sober. We had a good time. We talked.

We were watching TV one day and a commercial came on about coffins. An average sized coffin was $10,000. Some were made of satin, the Cadillac of coffins had everything in it, including a radio. "What the hell is that for?" I said, then joked to mom, "No damn way we're buying you one of those. We'll make one out of plywood and two-by-fours." Then the man on the TV said, "Now for those on the cheap end, there's this for $3,000." It was just a cardboard coffin. We were laughing. My whole family was like that. You could talk about it and still giggle about it. We said, "We could put you in a gunny sack and put you outside and put some plants around you and you could grow the plants," and we'd laugh some more. We were able to talk about something we knew was going to happen and deal with it. Before she passed, my mom would say, "I want you to have this picture," or "Don't forget this ring." She said, "I don't want to be buried with anything. Give things back and don't fight over anything. You see some of those families that fight, don't do that." So, we did as she wished. It was good. Being able to talk was good.

So, I lost my mom, my stepdad, and my sister Ruby Ann to cancer. Then a couple of years ago my grandson got taken to the hospital. That same night he and his mom were on a medevac to Edmonton. I went over to my son's house and sat with him. A few hours later the doctor said it was a tumour, and they had to operate in the morning. It was benign but that was really scary. I was so thankful. Everybody in our family gets a two-year check-up for colon cancer. We all check our kids for leukaemia and have regular check-ups to make sure they are healthy.

Nowadays, I help patients from the community and travel with them as their medical escort. I support people when they are being diagnosed. I sit with them in silence. There are people who are just floored when they find out they have cancer. They can't function. Some people don't remember going back to Larga, or being on the plane back home, or even greeting their family after they have been diagnosed.

I remember one time when I was little, the whole family had to go get checked at the hospital. They wanted to take my blood, and I didn't want to let them. Nobody explained why, and that was that. Years later I thought, "Oh my God, what if they were checking to have a bone marrow transplant for my sister and I never let them? What if I could have saved her life and I didn't?" That's why if anything happens, I try to tell people everything. I say, "These are the risks, the pros and cons."

Our Inuvik Cancer Support group gives hope. It's somewhere safe. When community members of all ages come together to share their cancer stories, they bond with one another and feel at ease talking about what they are going through. It's a safe space where people can talk to each other. Feelings are feelings, and it doesn't matter what type of cancer you have. Learning and talking to other people about it helps. It's a relief for people to be able to cry without shame. Sometimes people with cancer don't want to say they are not doing okay because they worry about the other person's feelings. Whenever we meet as a group, we feel a connection: the friendship and common battle bring us together.

When the World Indigenous Cancer Conference was held in Calgary in 2019, Agnes Pascal, Mary Roland, and I went to represent the Inuvik Cancer Support Group and the Northwest Territories. There were people there from around the world and no other people could say they had our type of little grassroots group in their country. The people at the conference were impressed with our group and that it was just for people who wanted to talk. They said they wanted to start their own group at home. I was so proud.

I would really like the doctors and nurses to talk about the fact that if you have cancer, you should stop sugar. Did we have cancer before there was sugar in our communities? Processed food and sugar are causing cancer. A lot of cancers can be cured nowadays. By learning more about cancer, the people working on it will eventually find a cure. I think if Ruby Ann had cancer today, she would probably be cured.

In terms of having a medical escort, it's important that the patient is comfortable with their escort knowing their personal information. There should be cancer advocates who can escort people who don't have anyone. Larga should be able to offer a cancer advocate to be there when a patient gets their results. Goba Care is like a patient advocate and could do that work as well, being with Northern patients at their doctors' appointments. I have never met the NWT cancer navigators. I've phoned and left a message. They are all located in Yellowknife but they should come to the communities too.

If you have cancer, it's important to have someone to talk to. Write down how you are doing, especially if you are being counted on by your family to be the caregiver. You have to have that spot in the house or outside where you go with your cup of tea or coffee and sit there and relax and breathe and take care of yourself in peace and quiet for the moment. Let bygones be bygones with people. You need to have a fresh start with people. Find people you can rely on when you are feeling all alone in the world.

I always believe life goes on, if not here on earth, your essence is somewhere else. Get things done while you're here. Go for holidays. Make memories and live life to the best so that the living can remember you when you're gone.

Clara Bates

TUKTOYAKTUK

I am 66 years old. I had colon cancer about sixteen years ago. I was very, very, very sick for three years. I had very bad pain in my lower back. Before I was diagnosed, I kept going to the health centre for three years complaining of symptoms with no help at all. I was losing a lot of weight. My hair was falling out. I was getting very weak. The health centre kept sending me home telling me that I was going to be okay. Three times I approached my MLA, the third time I went into his office and told him, "I am going to the CBC reporters and all the reporters and make it public that I've been going to the nursing station and no one is helping me with my pain, if you don't do something." After that the MLA contacted the minister of health and two days later, I was in the hospital under the knife. A month later I was told that I had colon cancer and that it was as big as the tip of my finger but that they took it out.

When the doctor told me I had cancer I asked, "Why didn't you tell me right away?" I was shocked but I also knew I had cancer well before they told me I did. I felt very angry with the health centre but at least I finally found out. My family was very shocked and grateful that the cancer was taken out. After the surgery I concentrated on trying to get better but I couldn't get better. I kept going to the health clinic because I couldn't stomach any kind of store-bought food. I tried to keep my house clean, but I was still very weak and realized I had to concentrate on my health more than on having a clean house. So, I concentrated on getting better. I must have gone down to 90 pounds. I couldn't even open a pop bottle. I could only drink caribou broth and sometimes eat fish.

During those years I was so sick that every time I looked out my window or went for a walk, I would see ancient faces in the ground all over. My friend said that her dad saw the same thing. I realized that our ancestors are in the ground watching us. I was sick and dying at that time, and everywhere I looked I was seeing visions of old ancient Inuit all over my community. I thought I was going crazy. I think when we are just about dying, we have extra vision. Our ancestors are with us. They are camouflaged.

During that time, my son asked me to adopt one of his daughters but I told him I couldn't adopt her because I was so sick. That really hurt me because I dreamed about the baby before she was born. I knew this little person was somebody special. My daughter was just turning 18 and she cried and cried for three months to adopt the baby. I kept telling my daughter she can't adopt her; she had to finish her education. But she wouldn't stop crying and sobbing and asking to adopt the baby. She said if I don't take the baby someone else will, so we adopted her. I rubbed rocks all over her body and we made sure our teardrops fell on her. I prayed that God would make her kind and helpful and now my granddaughter is 13 years old. She's wise like an old woman. I think she was sent to help me during that time. She always came to have tea with me. She lives in Yellowknife now with her mom. My daughter is really kind and loving. All my kids are. I taught them about being kind and grateful.

Even after we adopted my grandchild, I was still so sick that I didn't know how to get better. I went back to the health centre, and they sent me out for another operation. They took five lumps out of my large intestine, but they were not cancerous. After they took them out, I started getting better. I started gaining weight and started feeling like my normal self again. It was a real struggle though. I had to go through income support after I had to quit working. It was then that I started making Pangnirtung hats.[1] I had been crocheting for forty years. Now I make Pangnirtung hats for tourists. I make toques out of muskox wool too.

There were a couple other people who had cancer too during the time that I was sick. People were going to the health centre for years and just being sent home. So, me and this older lady who had cancer complained and took action.

My father died of cancer very slowly but we took care of him really well. When he died, I read the history of the DEW Line.[2] He got hired to help build the site. The non-Indigenous people were wearing moon suits and burying mercury and other contaminants. The Indigenous Peoples were working there but they were not wearing moon suits and burying contaminants. After reading the documents I realized that maybe that's where my father got cancer from. We lived not too far from the DEW Line and my father had a fishnet there.

My brothers and sisters are all in our 50s and 60s now and we are all pretty healthy. We abstain from alcohol. We have a big family. All my friends and relatives were calling me every day telling me they were praying for me. It went on for a good six months where people were calling and saying they were praying for me. I make sure I have a close connection with my family. We are a praying family. There's always hope for people.

There are so many people starting to get cancer, even the young people in our community. I think it is because we are relying more on store-bought food, because of contamination, because we are not living off the land anymore, and a lot of people are starting to smoke a lot now. All our lives we lived off the land and that's what made us strong. We hardly had store-bought meat. I was the main cook, being the oldest. We'd go spring hunting for a month. Living off the land made us so strong and so good. The food is there for us on the land to make us strong and healthy. From when I was very small, I learned how to scale a fish and cut up a ptarmigan or goose. Being on this earth and living in Tuk for many years I see that the fish were once really white and in the last few years they are a little darker, they have turned greyish. I'm wondering what is going on with our ocean. We live off the ocean.

For a long time, I was a single mother taking care of my three sons. I took a couple of courses and worked in an office for many years drinking coffee all day long. I got hooked on Coca-Cola but then I became allergic to it. I think that gave me colon cancer. The cancer could come back but I don't have to go to the doctor until I start feeling it come back. I watch myself really carefully.

The people who lived the longest in Tuk were the people that walked every day. I told myself I'm going to walk every day too and go for fresh air. I live alone now. I can clean my house now. I haven't had a drink for twenty-three years. I smoke weed though once in a while; it helps. I asked the doctor for medical cannabis but they did not give me a prescription. I had to deal with a lot of depression for a while. I had to be strong and go day by day. My three sons did not want to see me so sick. They thought I might have been dying so they kind of stayed away. They were so scared. They loved me so much that they tried to detach themselves to try to heal themselves.

When my uncles and aunts and dad had cancer, I never heard them complain at all. I marvel at how strong and patient they were. A lot of people have died in this town but we have no people to talk to at all for mental health support. It's a very tough town to live in but I love my town. I'll never leave my town at all. I was not offered any health care support at all here once I was diagnosed with cancer. For the first two or three years I never had an escort to the hospital down South until I found out I was able to get one. I wasn't even referred to a helper when my daughter moved out. I had no counsellors. I had to work it through. I was so thankful for my relatives, who were calling me every day telling me they were praying for me. There's no support at all here in Tuk for cancer patients, and even for grieving people there is no support.

I am thankful that I am okay now. I am so thankful and grateful. I have a voice, and I can speak up for all people here. I speak my mind and give the government a hard time and changed a few things in Tuk. Cancer has taught me to be caring, loving, and kind. You don't know what other people are going through. I'm grateful that I'm able to see my two great-grandchildren now. I try to do my best. If someone I know has cancer, I show them love and give them encouragement. I offer prayer.

I fell through the ice twice when I was young and almost died. There were a lot of things that happened to me, but I know God and his angels have always been there. He's saved my life so many times that I know he's got something planned for me, so I use my voice to speak out and better the people of the Northwest Territories.

Notes

1. Pangnirtung or "Pang" hats are fitted and crocheted hats made of colourful wool, often with a tassel. They are named after the community that invented the style and where they are still made today.
2. The Distant Early Warning (DEW) Line was a Cold War era system of radar stations across the Arctic regions of Canada.

Anonymous

THE LAND

I was born on the land. The first few years of my life I grew up in a camp. In 1964 we were moved into the community and that's when I had to go to school. It was scary because I only knew my family and nobody else. I didn't know anyone. I didn't even know English. We only spoke our language. When I was growing up a lot of the teachings were based on respect. I learned how to speak English but I never forgot my language. When my mom got sick, we didn't understand what kind of sickness she had. Only years later after she died, we found out it was cancer but never knew what type it was. That was in the early 70s when we still had about one flight a month. They would take the patients out to the hospital in Edmonton.

I myself had to go to Edmonton on medical as just a little child. Sometimes I'd be there for six months. I remember the year my mom passed, I was 8 years old. I spent months as a child in the Charles Camsell Hospital. I remember going to the hospital, but I don't remember what they did.

I grew up in a big family. There were ten of us. Out of the ten of us there's just five of us left. The other five all died from different kinds of cancers one year after another. The most recent one is my niece. She just recently passed from a brain tumour and my late father died of a brain

---

A beach along the Arctic Ocean. Photo by Bernadette Binder.

tumour too. Two of my brothers died, one from lung cancer and one from thyroid cancer. My older sister died of pancreatic cancer in 2013. In 2017, my second older sister died with leukaemia because they found it too late. In the fall of 2020, my last brother died of two different types of cancer in his body. I was their main caregiver, and it was really hard, but what made it easier was that I worked in the community health department for fifteen years and my job was to look after palliative care. My husband went through cancer too. He was very angry and had to go for surgery during COVID. When he got medevacked we couldn't go with him. He had to go through it all by himself in the hospital.

I'm a survivor from two different types of cancer. First it was ovarian cancer, which they removed. Then I had colon cancer and I've been in remission since 2014. In January, I went for an MRI on my brain, and they found a tumour but I have no symptoms. I'm waiting to hear from a doctor. They said its benign. If it was full-term cancer I would have lost my vision, my hearing. Even with my colon cancer I never had any symptoms until they found it.

When I first got my diagnosis for cancer my first thought was that I don't want to leave my baby behind; he was only 3 years old when they removed my ovaries. He was too small. All my other kids were grown-up but he was a baby. It took a while, but I got through the first year after the surgery and got stronger again. A few years later I got appendicitis so that sent me to Yellowknife. If my appendix didn't burst, they would have never found colon cancer. When they diagnosed me with colon cancer I said to the doctors, "Whatever you're going to do, do it. If it will help me live a little bit longer, then do it." I explained to my family what procedures I would be going through. I didn't go through chemo. Surgery was the only option. When I looked after palliative patients it was really hard to explain to the families what the process and diagnoses were and how it was going to be to the end. That was the hardest part. I knew those people growing up.

I used to be so scared at first. I was so scared about leaving my kids behind. What would they do? How would they live their lives without their mom? So, I really fought against my fear. Not against the disease but against my fear. I was angry and bitter. When they first diagnosed me, I was angry, and it was because of my fear of leaving family behind and being so young then. Even though people were telling me to pray I would say, "You do it, I'm not doing it." Now I understand. Now I know that with modern technology they could do things to help you. Before that they didn't have an option. I think that's why so many Elders and young adults refused treatments. They were afraid because they don't understand it. It's not explained to them in an easier way. It's explained in long words. I was thankful that my former doctor was working, and I was able to sit down with him and ask him all kinds of questions and he explained everything to me in a way that I could understand it. I thought, that's how it should be explained to everyone, because not being able to understand is what brought the fear.

But in the back of my mind, I was always scared about what I was going to go through. How am I going to leave people behind if I'm not ready? I told myself, "Okay, I will fight it, but I have to quit being angry and learn about it and teach it." When you carry trauma and heavy things it becomes your illness. Lately I've been thinking that I've carried so much that I don't speak about because growing up I was told, "Don't talk about those things to people," and for women it's worse. Now we are starting to open up. The things I hear nowadays from our Elders is that when you carry too much of the past it can become an illness, a chronic disease. So, don't be scared to talk about things that you are going through. I carried too much. That load you have goes through your body and sometimes you feel it.

Most of my support came from my workplace. I was still working; even after my surgeries I went right back to work. Every day in our morning meetings my colleagues would ask me, "Are you ready for your day? Have you left your fears at the door?" Now my outlook on this is completely different. The more I hear about people getting cancer the more I want to help support them, but they have to be the ones to say, "Help me." I'm slowly learning to open up to say, "I've gone through cancer more than once. Talk to your doctor, talk to your nurse, talk to your family. Don't just sit there in the corner in the dark and say, 'I'm going to die.'"

When I was growing up, the stories I heard from my late aunt and grandfather, they knew about cancer before anyone. They saw people who went from healthy to skin and bones and eventually die. They said no matter what they did to make them feel better they just got worse. Our Elders back then knew about cancer. Long ago they didn't have the doctors and nurses to help them, so people just did what they could to make them comfortable. Nowadays, even if you are diagnosed, especially the younger people, they lose it. They don't want to accept it. You have to explain that when you accept it, there is help. There are modern technologies.

When I was growing up, everything we ate was from the land. It was not contaminated. When we moved into the communities, there was more processed food and store-bought things and we stopped living off the land. I think that is what caused cancer. A few years after moving into the community people started to get sick. There's so much mercury put into canned goods that we didn't know about because we didn't know how to read. Alcohol and drugs came along and combined everything together and that's the scary part. What I always hear is when we lived off the land, we were so healthy. Our food was clean. We ate everything from the ground, from the ocean, from the lakes so we were always healthy. We never found animals with diseases like we do now. We don't do enough healthy activities. Back home I used to walk a lot. I still walk here but it's so cold, I don't walk far.

When I first got ovarian cancer, I went alone down South. Even though I was going through surgery they wouldn't allow me an escort. I had to go through everything alone and it was scary because I had nobody to be with me. The second time I went they said it was just a follow-up and I was scared then too. It's a good thing I had good friends that live in Yellowknife, and they are there for me. When I was diagnosed with colon cancer, I went by myself and went into surgery and I was alone. It was scary because there was nobody there to hold my hand, tell me everything will be okay and that I will get through it. You need somebody there to keep you going, to keep you strong. Even if it's just asking, "Are you in pain?" Even when I went for my MRI I went alone. I sat waiting for the results for two hours and I kept wondering why they didn't let anyone come with me. In a big city, you don't know anybody. You always need that support system with you. So many people get denied escorts, especially if they have to go for CT scans and MRI, and if they get diagnosed, they are all alone.

When I came home, I had no motivation to do anything. I didn't want to work, didn't want to see anyone. I stayed in my room. Didn't want to eat. I started to go into a depression for a while. I told my doctor what I was going through, and he reassured me that everything would be okay. He said, "Don't think of your family, of how they are going to suffer. Instead, think of how you are going to get through it."

When I told my family I was going for a CT scan I thought that I would be okay because I had been walking and eating healthy. One Elder I met in Yellowknife, she was from the Sahtu; she spoke only in her language. She would wheel past my room and wave at me. One day she came in with her escort, a young girl. She came into my room and held my hand and smiled at me. She touched my face. When she was leaving, she told her escort to tell me, "All good now." And they walked out of the room. A week later I was discharged, and I stayed with my friend who took care of me. For some reason I kept thinking of that Elder. Every day when I woke up I thought of her. Every time I thought of her, I felt better again. When she touched my hand, I could feel warmth. It's amazing. I don't even know her.

Every day my family would call and ask how I am. When I came home my kids gave me a lot of support. As soon as I woke up, they'd be beside me and make me something to eat. They would take me for a walk or bring me where I needed to go. They are so supportive. They supported me through my roughest time when I was losing a lot of family to cancer, and I couldn't get home to them because of what I was going through. Even to this day my children are always there for me even though they are grown. When I think about all the things I went through now and all the support I had, I kind of regret not telling my kids that they need to have their own support system too.

My family from back home checks up on me every week, and every day I get a message from my nieces and nephews. I get a lot of support from my friends too. The majority of my friends are sober. I don't drink. I still smoke cigarettes. When I first came home out of my surgery they came and visited me and asked me if I needed anything. After I had my surgery and was in the hospital I couldn't stay in bed. I asked someone to bring me food because all they were giving me was Jell-O and tea. Now I can't stand Jell-O. Even to this day my friends still call me and ask me how I am and if I need anything. Once a month me and my friend go out on the highway. Sometimes I go out there and scream my head off and cry.

Lots of young people at home are losing their families from cancer. Most of these young people are so angry. They really need to be informed, the younger generations. Many of them, as soon as they are diagnosed, they turn to alcohol and drugs because they are afraid. If you have to go to treatment you have to go down South and leave everyone behind. If they had a healing centre here it would be so much easier because then a whole family could be involved, and you could do a gathering. You could ask how they feel about their family member being sick and what they could do to deal with it or get more support instead of sending one person away. How are other family members supposed to know what they are going through? A lot of the times I see that happening and the family turns to alcohol and drugs, and when the person gets home there's no support.

I have a counsellor I see each week. I talk to her about how I feel, what I'm going through. And she's always supporting me. She reassures me. When I'm alone in the evenings sometimes I find myself crying out of nowhere. Then I think to myself, "What am I doing?" I almost slip down into depression, and I say, "I can't do that. I have lots of life yet. I can get through it." I push myself. I was given a chance to stay in this world after overcoming two different types of cancer. If I have to fight to the end, I'll fight to the end until I'm done.

Cancer brought my family closer. We are closer now more than ever even though we are living far away from one another. I have a lot of support at work. The women I work with helped me through that first year after I was diagnosed. Financially they made sure I was on top of my bills. They put me on medical leave, but after four months I said I'm going back. That's what kept me going, work. I pushed myself to get up every day and go to work. The support system I have there is so good for me. I do medical interpreting for the hospital. I did it voluntarily for the first few years. They hired me because I could speak the three language dialects of our area. But even interpreters need a support system.

I have a new beginning. I've got a roof over my head. I've got food. I'm still here. I can do it. It's getting better. When I get up in the morning I say, "Thank you, I'm here, I'm awake, I can do things." At the end of the day, I say thanks for the whole day. I never say I'm going to do this tomorrow or the next day. I just go day by day. The way I was raised was to respect myself and everyone else around me. I am slowly telling myself now that I have to start doing things for me for a change. Everything I do is for everybody else. Sometimes when I don't want to say no, I have to say no.

Look for somebody that you trust, somebody that you are close to that you can open up to. Somebody you are comfortable with. Someone that's not going to tell anyone else unless they get your permission first. I really have to learn to do things for me more to make me feel better. Not because I don't want to do things for other people but because my kids are all grown up and I can do the things I want to do. I'm not going to go sailing around the world, but I will give more support to myself so that I can have the time and energy to help others. Even if it's really cold out, I just take a short little walk. When I come home the kids say, "Did you finish your me time?" I'm learning. It's a struggle. You just have to take it step by step. I'm just going to take my time and work on myself. I got through the worst parts and now I can deal with it. I got the support system I need.

Advice and Actions
FROM *BOOK OF HOPE* STORYTELLERS

The following pages contain advice and actions drawn from the experiences shared by the contributors to this book. There is guidance for medical professionals, decision makers, and policy professionals within health systems, caregivers of cancer patients, and for cancer patients themselves. While some things are specific to a Northern context, many are relevant beyond that.

Advice for Medical Professionals

- Good communication is essential — communicate clearly and thoroughly with patients about their diagnosis and treatment. Make sure information is provided about what to expect.
- Do not delay giving a diagnosis of cancer, ever.
- Do not make assumptions about what a patient knows, and be upfront and totally honest with the patient.
- Provide resources and support in advance — before someone has surgery and starts treatment.
- Cultivate a caring and compassionate attitude with all patients; your words and actions really matter to patients.
- Educate yourself and your colleagues about what life is like for Northerners who have to go South for medical care and how you can make it more comfortable for patients.

Actions for Decision Makers and Policy Professionals

- Take immediate action to understand why so many Northerners are not diagnosed with cancer sooner even when they have accessed health care services multiple times with symptoms.

- Currently the system requires patients to advocate for themselves and their needs. This is not equitable, as not everyone has the knowledge or experience to know how to advocate. *Professional supports and advocates should be available for everyone who needs them.*
- Medical escorts are essential for all patients with cancer or facing a potential cancer diagnosis. No one should be alone when receiving a diagnosis of cancer. Everyone needs support, and escorts can help to take notes, bring joy and laughter, and be there when a person weeps or admits they are scared. *All cancer patients should be offered an escort without question.*
- Cancer patients need someone to talk to, and they often don't want to worry their family and friends. There should be dedicated mental health support for cancer patients at every stage of their journey
  » Cancer patients need to connect with others who have had cancer through cancer sharing circles or other peer support networks in person or virtually/over the phone. Women, men, and children may need their own groups.
  » Elders can provide support to cancer patients too.
  » Caregivers, family, and friends also need emotional support. This includes the children of cancer patients.
- Implement changes to make medical travel less of a financial and emotional burden for patients and their families.
- Limit the administrative burden of accessing care: many patients find this overwhelming.
- Feed patients well at hospitals — provide tasty, nourishing, and culturally appropriate food.
- Educate doctors and front-line health workers about what life is like for Northerners who have to go South for medical care and how they can make it more comfortable for patients.
- Consider the impact of overlapping emergencies on those with cancer — for example, the isolation requirements of the COVID-19 pandemic added additional stress to an already difficult time for patients.
- More information about cancer and cancer prevention needs to be provided to Northerners.
- Make sure resources are available and accessible in small communities and not just in Yellowknife or regional centres.

- Support traditional Indigenous economies and access to country foods and medicines for good health.

Advice for Caregivers

- Recognize that someone who has just been diagnosed with cancer probably feels like their world is turning upside down.
- Often, just being there is enough; sometimes people don't want to talk.
- If someone facing a cancer diagnosis wants to talk, let them talk because storytelling is healing.
- Encourage them to cry if they need to. Crying is medicine.
- Ask the person if they need a hug. Stop and listen and invite them to share whatever they need to. Show that you care.
- Realize that even if you want to fix it for them, you can't.
- Never tell people with cancer they're going to be okay because it's not possible to know what will happen.
- Don't tell someone with cancer to be strong or to stay positive.
- If it feels appropriate, consider giving a cancer patient a cookbook designed for cancer patients, so they have ideas about healthy food to put in their bodies. You can prepare and share healthy food with them, too.
- Don't force anything onto someone with cancer that they're not ready for. Always go at their pace.
- Certain types of treatment and chemo fatigue can cause patients to be grumpy, and cancer itself can cause many to feel insecure or anxious. Be aware that the character and mood of cancer patients may change. Be patient and don't take it personally.
- Offer to support someone with cancer or to help find someone else to support them.
- When appropriate, offer faith and prayer. Let them know God is with them and to have faith, and offer to pray with them.
- Provide the person with helpful resources and information about what to expect.
- Share your own journey with cancer if you have one.
- Try to help them find happiness and hope and throw in a few laughs too. Laughter is also medicine.

Advice for Cancer Patients

- Watch for anything concerning and get it checked. If cancer screening is available to you, get screened.
- When you first get diagnosed, get grounded. Take some deep breaths and sit with it. You'll take it one step at a time.
- When you are ready, reach out to those around you. People will want to help, and you'll need support around you.
- Try to have different kinds of support around you. Cancer survivors in this book benefited from support of friends and family as well as from people who have been through cancer or were going through it at the same time.
- Don't be scared to talk about the things that you are going through. Talk to your doctor, talk to your nurse, talk to your family and friends, talk to other cancer patients.
- Look for ways to deepen your faith, if that feels right to you. Many storytellers in this book benefited from this.
- Whenever you struggle with emotions, work on finding peace (whatever this looks like for you).
- Advocate for yourself and be persistent when dealing with the medical system. Ask for help to advocate if you need it.
- Do your research and learn as much as you can about what you're going through. Don't depend on doctors to be your teachers; learn on your own and have someone help you if you need it.
- Expect to have an escort for medical travel, and do not accept not having one. It is not up to medical travel; it is up to you and your doctor. Whoever you are and whatever stage of your cancer journey you are at, you deserve someone with you to help with listening to information, taking notes, asking questions, discussing what oncologists and other specialists say after appointments, and being there for you however you need them to be.
- Find a way to keep track of all the documents and appointments and reports and bring them with you to appointments. Things you will want to bring with you include: family medical history, medications, a calendar for appointment dates, and copies of pathologist reports.

- Ask questions. Write them down to bring with you to appointments.
- Use traditional medicine like spruce gum if that feels right to you. But if you are going to gather medicine yourself, make sure you know the proper protocol.
- Know that this whole experience is making you stronger.
- Have hope and don't give up!

Acknowledgements

My heartfelt thank you, mahsi cho, to each and every one of the contributors to this book. Thank you for sharing your stories and trusting me with them.

During a presentation about the Inuvik Cancer Support Group, I mentioned the idea of the *Book of Hope* out loud for the first time in public. Afterwards, Crystal Milligan invited me to meet with her to discuss it. Crystal ran with the idea and secured funding from Hotıì ts'eeda to begin our interviews with storytellers. Katłıà Lafferty and Sara Komarnisky helped to bring this book over the finish line. I can't thank these ladies enough.

I also want to thank others who have supported this project, including Amanda Chaulk-Parrott, Jullian MacLean, Stephanie Irlbacher-Fox, Danita Frost-Arey, Holly Hesk Jones, members of the Inuvik Cancer Support Group, Aurora College, Kristian Binder, Tony Devlin, Fazeela Jiwa, Lauren Jeanneau, Brenda Conroy and everyone at Fernwood Publishing, Hotıì ts'eeda, Government of the Northwest Territories, and Gwich'in Tribal Council. Thank you to Heidi Scarfone for the beautiful prints presented to *Book of Hope* storytellers.

This book is a tribute to David Malcolm — a dear friend and inspiration for this book. I first heard David and Sandra's story during a one-time cancer sharing circle in Inuvik. Their story was emotionally overwhelming to me as a listener, but they displayed a beautiful inner peace as they shared it. David spoke of his illness in a way that helps others to see what it really is like to live with cancer. Then with that same breath, he would share his faith and hope. He was an amazing man who shared with such humbleness. On behalf of the Inuvik Cancer Support Group, thank you David for allowing us to be a part of your journey.

Two close friends experienced the same type of cancer that I did: Ister (Velma) Frost and Roseanne Francis. I remember how sad I felt when they were diagnosed. I wasn't sure what type of support they needed. But when I was diagnosed with cancer, I contacted these two ladies right away. God placed these two angels to guide me through the toughest and scariest time of my life. They explained radiation and chemotherapy to me. When I cried at the thought of losing my hair, they shared their own experiences and encouraged me to move forward. These friends helped me build the endurance I needed to persevere by telling me what's going to happen next. If I can offer support to others as shown to me by these two, I would be grateful. Mahsi Ister and Roseanne.

I want to thank my home community of Fort McPherson and everyone throughout the Northwest Territories for all your support and prayers, including my Uncle Neil Pascal, my Auntie Mary Effie Snowshoe, and my parents Martha and Winston Moses. Mahsi for your encouragement and all the love shown to me and my children. My blessings to Ronnie, Laura, and Seanna Pascal, who are my biggest inspiration in life. Thank you for your love and understanding. My jijuu Laura, this is for you from your shibeebii (baby), forever in my heart.